TNM Atlas

Illustrated Guide to the TNM/pTNM Classification

of Malignant Tumours

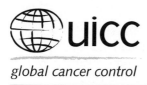

global cancer control

TNM Atlas

Illustrated Guide to the
TNM/pTNM Classification of Malignant Tumours

5th Edition 2005

Editors
Ch. Wittekind, F.L. Greene, R.V.P. Hutter,
M. Klimpfinger and L.H. Sobin

With 505 illustrations
and an insert with summaries
of the T and N definitions by site

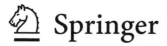

Prof. Dr. Ch. Wittekind
Direktor des Instituts für Pathologie
Universität Leipzig
Liebigstr. 26
D-04103 Leipzig

Dr. F. L. Greene
Carolinas Medical Center
Department of Surgery
1000 Blythe Boulevard
Charlotte, NC 28203, USA

Dr. R. V. P. Hutter
30 Surrey Lane
Livingston, HJ 07039, USA

Dr. L. H. Sobin
Division of Gastrointestinal
and Hepatic Pathology
Armed Forces Institute of Pathology
Washington, DC 20306, USA

Prof. Dr. M. Klimpfinger
Vorstand des Pathologischen
und bakteriologischen Instituts
Kaiser-Franz-Josef-Spital
Kundratstrasse 3
A-1110 Vienna

2nd printing, corrected 2007

ISBN-13   978-3-540-44234-9   5th edition   Springer-Verlag   Berlin   Heidelberg   New York
ISBN-13   978-3-540-63799-8   4th edition   Springer-Verlag   Berlin   Heidelberg   New York

Bibliographic information Deutsche Bibliothek
Die Deutsche Bibliothek lists this publication in the Deutsche Nationalbibliografie;
detailed bibliographic data is available in the Internet at <http://dnb.ddb.de>.

Springer is a part of Springer Science+Business Media

springer.com

© Springer-Verlag Berlin Heidelberg 2005

Printed in Germany

Planing: Ulrike Conrad-Willmann
Project management: Lindrum Weber
Cover design: deblik, Berlin
Illustrations: Peter Lübke, Wachenheim, Germany
Typesetting: Satz-Druck-Service, 69181 Leimen, Germany
Printed on acid-free paper   106/2111 – 5 4 3 2   SPIN 12211012

Contents

Preface to the Fifth Edition

This new fifth edition of the TNM Atlas reflects the changes in the TNM System introduced by the recently published 6th edition of the TNM Classification of Malignant Tumours [1]. The most important additions and modifications are:

- A revised classification of head and neck tumours reflecting the introduction of T4a/pT4a and T4b/pT4b categories, which allow a ramification in locally operable and non operable tumours
- A new classification of tumours of the nasal cavity
- Changes in the classification of thyroid tumours
- New subcategories in the classification of gastric tumours
- Changes in the classifications of tumours of the liver, gallbladder, extrahepatic bile ducts, liver
- A new classification of malignant mesothelioma of pleura
- Changes in the classification of bone tumours
- Substantial changes in the classification of malignant melanoma of the skin
- Changes in the classification of regional lymph nodes of the breast
- Modifications in the definition of risk factors of gestational trophoblastic tumours according to the proposals of FIGO
- New subcategories in the classification of tumours of the prostate
- Changes in the classifications of ophthalmic tumours

Additionally, a proposal for the classification of sentinel lymph nodes was introduced as well as a classification of isolated tumour cells (ITC) in regional lymph nodes and bone marrow.

The editorial board has changed: Dr. Hermanek, the editor-in-chief of the former edition and one of the "fathers" of the TNM Atlas, has retired, as has Dr. Wagner; Dr. Klimpfinger has joined the board. The editors wish to express many thanks to Paul Hermanek for his great contributions to the development and promotion of the TNM Atlas and to Dr. Wagner for his valuable work.

The editorial board has tried to follow the innovative concept developed by Bernd Spiessl to provide a graphic aid for the practical application of the TNM classification system. The TNM classification, as presented and illustrated in this edition, corresponds exactly to the 6th edition of the UICC TNM Classification of Malignant Tumours [1] and the 6th edition of the AJCC Cancer Staging Manual [2]. Recent modifications by FIGO [3] are also included in order to keep the FIGO and TNM classifications identical.

Substantial changes between the revised fourth edition (1998) and the present edition of the TNM Atlas are indicated by a line at the left-hand side of the page.

The editors hope that the TNM Atlas will continue to facilitate the daily practice of oncologists and to enhance the use of TNM in planning treatment, estimating prognosis and evaluating treatment results.

Ch. Wittekind, Leipzig
F. L. Greene, Charlotte, NC
R. V. P. Hutter, Livingston, NJ
M. Klimpfinger, Vienna
L.H. Sobin, Washington, DC

April 2004

References

1. UICC: TNM Classification of Malignant Tumours. 6th edition (2002). Sobin LH, Wittekind Ch (eds). Wiley, New York
2. Greene FL, Balch CM, Fleming ID, Fritz A, Haller DG, Morrow M, Page DL (eds) (2002) AJCC cancer staging manual, 6th edn. Springer, New York
3. Creasman WT, Odicino F, Maisoneuve P, Beller U, Benedet JL, Heintz APM, Ngan HYS, Sideri M, Pecorelli S (2001) FIGO Annual report on the results and treatment in gynaecological cancer, vol 24. Carcinoma of the corpus uteri. J Epidemiol Biostat 6:45–86

Foreword to the First Edition

Confronted with a myriad of T's, N's and M's in the UICC TNM booklet, classifying a malignancy may seem to many cancer clinicians a tedious, dull and pedantic task. But with a look at the TNM Atlas all of a sudden lifeless categories become vivid images, challenging the clinicians's know-how and investigational skills.

Brigit van der Werf-Messing, M. D.
Professor of Radiology
Chairman of the International TNM-Committee of the UICC

Rotterdam, July 1982

Acknowledgements

The editors wish to express their thanks to Prof. Dr. Dr. h. c. Paul Hermanek, Erlangen, for his invaluable help in the preparation of the manuscript and illustrations.

They are equally grateful to Mr. P. Lübke who took great care in drawing the anatomical illustrations.

Funding of the TNM Project by the Centers for Disease Control and Prevention (USA) through grant HR3/CCH417470 is gratefully acknowledged. The content of the publication is solely the responsibility of the authors and do not necessarily represent the official views of the CDC.

Finally the Editors wish to thank Springer-Verlag and staff for their expertise.

Editors

Prof. Dr. Ch. Wittekind
Direktor des Institutes für Pathologie
Universität Leipzig
Liebigstr. 26
D-04103 Leipzig

Dr. F. L. Greene
Carolinas Medical Center
Department of Surgery
1000 Blythe Boulevard
Charlotte, NC 28203, USA

Dr. R. V. P. Hutter
30 Surrey Lane
Livingston, HJ 07039, USA

Dr. L.H. Sobin, Professor of Pathology
Head, Division of Gastrointestinal
Pathology
Armed Forces Institute of Pathology
Washington, DC 20306, USA

Professor Dr. M. Klimpfinger
Vorstand des Pathologischen
und bakteriologischen Institutes
Kaiser-Franz-Josef-Spital
Kundratstrasse 3
A-1110 Wien

Contributors to the Fifth Edition

Bootz, F., Bonn, FRG	Head and Neck Surgery
Hermanek, P., Erlangen, FRG	Pathology
Sobin, L.H., Washington/DC, USA	Pathology
Spraul, Ch., Ulm, FRG	Ophthalmology
Weber, Anette, Leipzig, FRG	Head and Neck Surgery
Wittekind, Ch., Leipzig, FRG	Pathology

Contributors to the Fourth Edition

Bootz, F., Leipzig, FRG	Head and neck surgery
Hermanek, P., Erlangen, FRG	Pathology
Howaldt, H.-P., Gießen, FRG	Head and neck surgery
Hutter, R.V.P., Livingstone/NJ, USA	Pathology
Paterok, E., Erlangen, FRG	Gynaecology
Sobin, L.H., Washington/DC, USA	Pathology
Wagner, G., Heidelberg, FRG	Documentation and Epidemiology
Wittekind, Ch., Leipzig, FRG	Pathology

Contributors to the Third Edition

Baker, H. W., Portland, Ore, USA — Head and neck surgery
Beahrs, O. H., Rochester, Minn, USA — General surgery
Drepper, H., Münster-Handorf, FRG — Maxillofacial surgery
Gemsenjäger, E., Basel, Switzerland — General surgery
Genz, T., Berlin — Gynaecology
Glanz, H., Marburg, FRG — Otorhinolaryngology
Hasse, J., Freiburg, FRG — Thoracic surgery
Hermanek, P., Erlangen, FRG — Pathology
Hutter, R. V. P., Livingston, NJ, USA — Pathology
Kindermann, G., München, FRG — Gynaecology
Kleinsasser, O., Marburg, FRG — Otorhinolaryngology
Lang, G., Erlangen, FRG — Ophthalmology
Naumann, G. O. H., Erlangen, FRG — Ophthalmology
Remagen, W., Basel, Switzerland — Pathology
Scheibe, O., Stuttgart, FRG — General surgery
Schmitt, H. P., Heidelberg, FRG — Neuropathology
Sobin, L. H., Washington, DC, USA — Pathology
Spiessl, B., Basel, Switzerland — Maxillofacial surgery
Wagner, G., Heidelberg, FRG — Documentation and Epidemiology

Contributors to the Second Edition

Adolphs, H. D., Höxter, FRG	Urology
Amberger, H., Heidelberg, FRG	General surgery
Baumann, R. P., Neuchâtel, Switzerland	Pathology
Berger, H., Göttingen, FRG	Dermatology
Bokelmann, D., Essen, FRG	General surgery
Brandeis, W. F., Heidelberg, FRG	Paediatric oncology
Dold, U., Gauting, FRG	Internal medicine
Drepper, H., Münster-Handorf, FRG	Maxillofacial surgery
Drings, P., Heidelberg, FRG	Internal medicine
Gemsenjäger, E., Basel, Switzerland	General surgery
Hasse, J., Basel, Switzerland	Thoracic surgery
Heitz, Ph., Basel, Switzerland	Pathology
Hermanek, P., Erlangen, FRG	Pathology
Karrer, K., Wien, Austria	Oncological epidemiology
Kuehnl-Petzold, C. Freiburg i.Br., FRG	Dermatology
Liebenstein, J., Mannheim, FRG	Gynaecology
Molitor, D., Bonn, FRG	Urology
Nidecker, A., Basel, Switzerland	Radiology
Rohde, H., Köln FRG	General surgery
Scheibe, O., Stuttgart, FRG	General surgery
Schmitt, A., Mannheim, FRG	Gynaecology
Spiessl, B., Basel, Switzerland	Maxillofacial surgery
Thomas, C., Marburg, FRG	Pathology
Vogt-Moykopf, I., Heidelberg, FRG	Thoracic surgery
Wagner, G., Heidelberg, FRG	Documentation and Epidemiology

Preliminary Note[1]

The TNM system for describing the anatomical extent of disease is based an the assessment of three components:

T – The extent of the primary tumour
N – The absence or presence and extent of regional lymph node metastasis
M – The absence or presence of distant metastasis

The addition of numbers to these three components indicates the extent of the malignant disease, thus:

T0, T1, T2, T3, T4; N0, N1, N2, N3; M0, M1

In effect, the system is a "shorthand notation" for describing the extent of a particular malignant tumour.

Each site is described under the following headings:
1. *Anatomy.*
   Drawings of the anatomical sites and subsites are presented with the appropriate ICD-O topography numbers.[1]
2. *Regional Lymph Nodes.*
   The regional lymph nodes are listed and shown in drawings.
3. *T/pT Clinical and Pathological Classification of the Primary Tumour.*
   The definitions for T and pT categories are presented. In the sixth edition (2002) of the TNM Classification the clinical and pathological classification (T and pT) generally coincide, therefore the same illustrations are valid for the T and pT classification. The only exception to this are malignant melanoma of conjunctiva and uvea, as well as retinoblastoma.
4. *N/pN Clinical and Pathological Classification of Regional Lymph Nodes.*
   The N and pN categories are presented in a fashion similar to the T and pT categories. Differences between N and pN definitions in the sixth edition arise only in the case of carcinoma of the breast and germ cell tumours of the testis.
5. *M/pM Clinical and Pathological Classification of Distant Metastasis.*
   M localization is given only in selected cases because of its many possible variables.

---

[1] ICD-O International Classification of Diseases for Oncology, 3rd edn (2000), WHO, Geneva

C Factor

The C factor, or certainty factor, reflects the validity of classification according to the diagnostic methods employed. Its use is optional.

The C factor definitions are:

C1 Evidence from standard diagnostic means (e.g., inspection, palpation and standard radiography, intraluminal endoscopy for tumours of certain regions)

C2 Evidence obtained by special diagnostic means, e.g., radiographic imaging in special projections, tomography, computed tomography (CT), ultrasonography, lymphography, angiography; scintigraphy; magnetic resonance imaging (MRI); endoscopy, biopsy, and cytology

C3 Evidence from surgical exploration, including biopsy and cytology

C4 Evidence of the extent of disease following definitive surgery and pathological examination of the resected specimen

C5 Evidence from autopsy

Example

Degrees of C may be applied to the T, N and M categories. A case might be described as T3C2, N2C1, M0C2.

The TNM clinical classification is, therefore, equivalent to C1, C2 and C3 in varying degrees of certainty, while the pTNM pathological classification generally is equivalent to C4.

Residual Tumour (R) Classification

The absence or presence of residual tumour after treatment should be described by the symbol R.

TNM and pTNM describe the anatomical extent of cancer in general without considering treatment. They can be supplemented by the R classification, which deals with tumour status after treatment. The R classification reflects the effects of therapy, influences further therapeutic procedures and is a strong predictor of prognosis.

In the R classification, not only local-regional residual tumour is to be taken into consideration, but also distant residual tumour in the form of remaining distant metastases.

The definitions of the R categories are:

RX Presence of residual tumour cannot be assessed
R0 No residual tumour (Fig. 1a-c)
RI Microscopic residual tumour (Fig. 2)
R2 Macroscopic residual tumour (Fig. 3a,b)

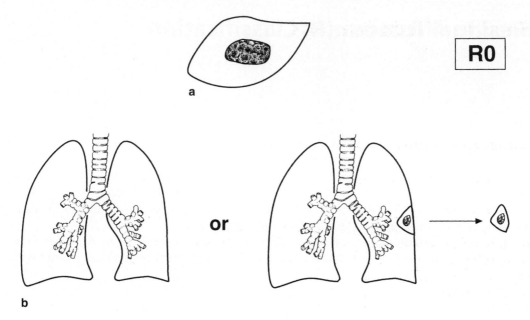

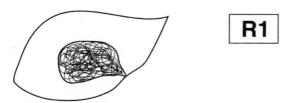

Fig. 1a–c. R0: **a** Primary tumour excised, resection margins without tumour. **b** No distant metastasis or distant metastasis completely removed.

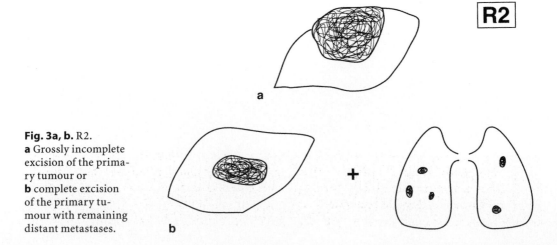

Fig. 2. R1. Excision of the primary tumour grossly complete, but histological examination demonstrates tumour at resection margins.

Fig. 3a, b. R2. **a** Grossly incomplete excision of the primary tumour or **b** complete excision of the primary tumour with remaining distant metastases.

Head and Neck Tumours

Introductory Notes

The following sites are included:

- Lip, oral cavity
- Pharynx: Oropharynx, nasopharynx, hypopharynx
- Larynx: Supraglottis, glottis, subglottis
- Maxillary sinus
- Nasal cavity, ethmoid sinus
- Salivary gland(s)
- Thyroid gland

Carcinomas arising in minor salivary glands of the upper aerodigestive tract are classified according to the rules for tumours of their anatomic site of origin, e.g., oral cavity.

Substantial changes in the 5th edition compared to the 4th edition are marked by a bar at the left-hand side of the page. The same is true for new classifications of previously unclassified tumours.

Regional Lymph Nodes (Fig. 4)

The definitions of the N categories for all head and neck sites except nasopharynx and thyroid are the same. These include:

(1)   submental nodes
(2)   submandibular nodes
(3)   cranial jugular (deep cervical) nodes
(4)   medial jugular (deep cervical) nodes
(5)   caudal jugular (deep cervical) nodes
(6)   dorsal cervical (superficial cervical) nodes along the accessory nerve
(7)   supraclavicular nodes
(8)   prelaryngeal, pretracheal* and paratracheal nodes
(9)   retropharyngeal nodes
(10)   parotid nodes
(11)   buccal nodes
(12)   retroauricular and occipital nodes

Note
* The pretracheal lymph nodes are sometimes addressed as "Delphian nodes".

N/pN Classification: Regional Lymph Nodes

The definitions of the N and pN categories for all head and neck sites except nasopharynx and thyroid gland are:

NX/pNX   Regional lymph nodes cannot be assessed
N/pNX   Regional lymph nodes cannot be assessed
N/pN0   No regional lymph nodes metastasis

pN0   Histological examination of a selective neck dissection specimen will ordinarily include 6 or more lymph nodes. Histological examination of a radical or modified radical neck dissection specimen will ordinarily include 10 or more lymph nodes. If the lymph nodes are negative, but the number ordinarily examined is not met, classify as pN0.
When the size is a criterion for pN classification, measurement is made of the metastasis, not of the entire lymph node.

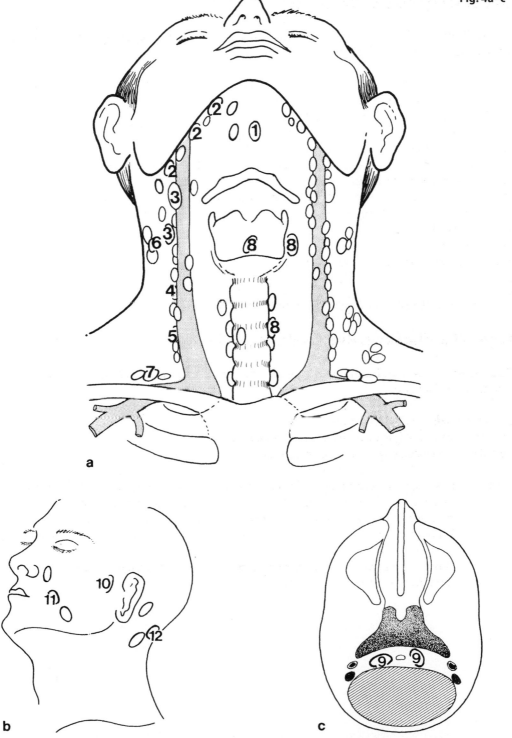

a

b

c

N1/pN1   Metastasis in a single ipsilateral lymph node, 3 cm or less in greatest dimension (Fig. 5)

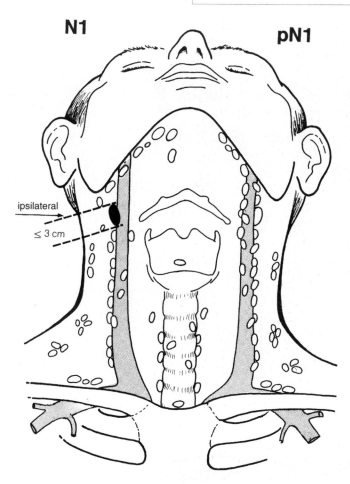

Any head or neck primary except nasopharynx and thyroid gland

Fig. 5

N1   **pN1**

ipsilateral

≤ 3 cm

N2/pN2   Metastasis in a single ipsilateral lymph node, more than 3 cm but not more than 6 cm in greatest dimension; or in multiple ipsilateral lymph nodes, none more than 6 cm in greatest dimension; or in bilateral or contralateral lymph nodes, none more than 6 cm in greatest dimension

  N2a/pN2a   Metastasis in a single ipsilateral lymph node,   more than 3 cm but not more than 6 cm in greatest dimension (Fig. 6)

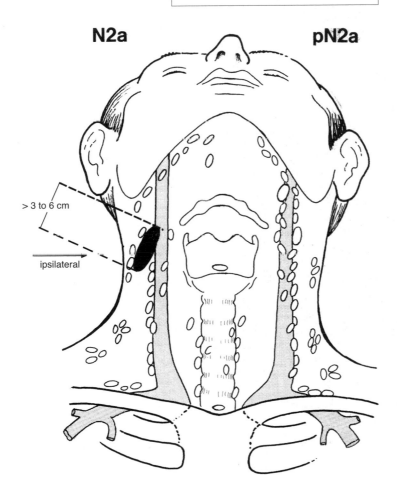

Fig. 6

Any head or neck primary except nasopharynx and thyroid gland

N2a

pN2a

> 3 to 6 cm

ipsilateral

Head and Neck Tumours

N2b/pN2b   Metastatsis in multiple ipsilateral lymph node, none more than 6 cm in greatest dimension (Fig. 7)

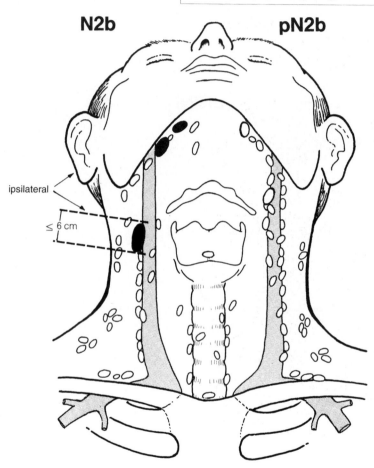

Fig. 7

N2c/pN2c   Metastasis in bilateral or contralateral lymph nodes, none more than 6 cm in greatest dimension (Fig. 8)

Fig. 8

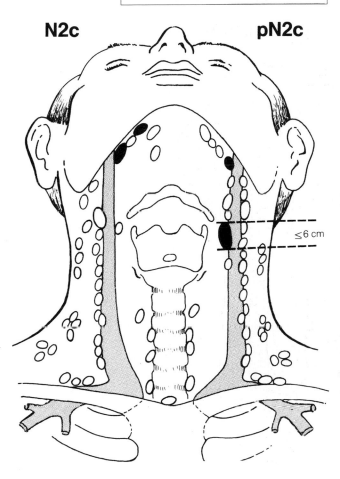

N3/pN3   Metastasis in a lymph node, more than 6 cm in greatest dimension (Fig. 9)

Note
Midline nodes are considered ipsilateral nodes.

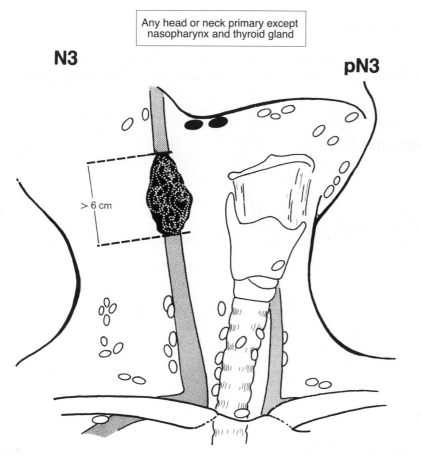

Any head or neck primary except nasopharynx and thyroid gland

N3

pN3

> 6 cm

Fig. 9

Lip and Oral Cavity (ICD-O C00, C02-C06)

Rules for Classification

The classification applies only to carcinomas of the vermilion surfaces of the lips and of the oral cavity, including those of minor salivary glands. There should be histological confirmation of the disease.

Anatomical Sites and Subsites

Lip (Fig.10)

1. External upper lip (vermilion border) (C00.0)
2. External lower lip (vermilion border) (C00.1)
3. Commissures (C00.6)

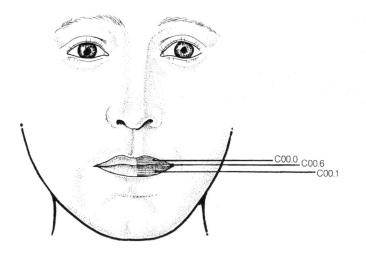

Fig. 10

C00.0 C00.6
C00.1

Oral Cavity (Figs. 11–13)

1. Buccal mucosa
   (i)   Mucosa of upper and lower lips (C00.3, 4)
   (ii) Cheek mucosa (C06.0)
   (iii) Retromolar areas (C06.2)
   (iv) Bucco-alveolar sulci, upper and lower (vestibule of mouth) (C06.1)
2. Upper alveolus and gingiva (upper gum) (C03.0)
3. Lower alveolus and gingiva (lower gum) (C03.1)
4. Hard palate (C05.0)
5. Tongue
   (i) Dorsal surface and lateral borders anterior to vallate papillae   (anterior two-thirds) (C02.0, 1)
   (ii) Inferior (ventral) surface (C02.2)
6. Floor of mouth (C04)

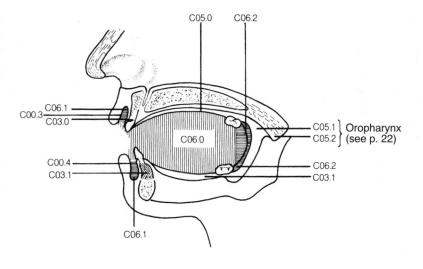

Fig. 11

Fig. 12

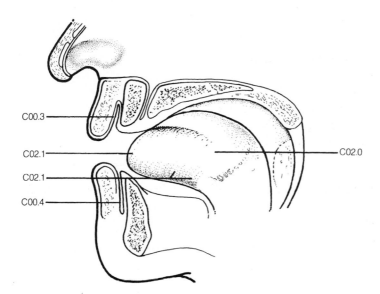

C00.3

C02.1

C02.1

C00.4

C02.0

Fig. 13

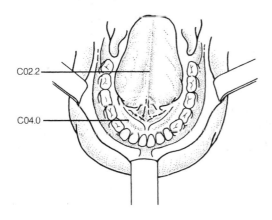

C02.2

C04.0

N- Regional Lymph Nodes

See p. 6/7.

TN Clinical Classification

T – Primary Tumour

TX   Primary tumour cannot be assessed
T0   No evidence of primary tumour
Tis   Carcinoma in situ

T1   Tumour 2 cm or less in greatest dimension (Figs. 14, 15)
T2   Tumour more than 2 cm but not more than 4 cm in greatest dimension (Figs. 16, 17)
T3   Tumour more than 4 cm in greatest dimension (Figs. 18, 19)

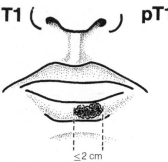

Fig. 14

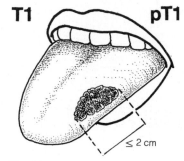

Fig. 15

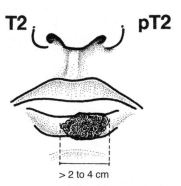

Fig. 16

T2   **pT2**   **Fig. 17**

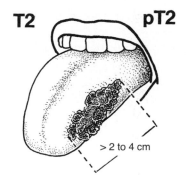

> 2 to 4 cm

T3 (   ) **pT3**   **Fig. 18**

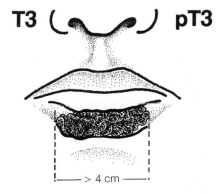

> 4 cm

T3   **pT3**   **Fig. 19**

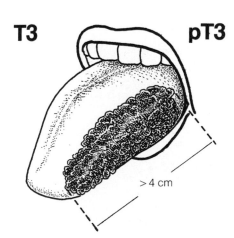

>4 cm

T4a   *Lip:* Tumour invades through cortical bone, inferior alveolar nerve, floor of mouth, or skin (chin or nose) (Figs. 20,21))

T4a   *Oral cavity:* Tumour invades through cortical bone, into deep/extrinsic muscle of tongue (genioglossus, hypoglossus, palatoglossus, and styloglossus), maxillary sinus, or skin of face (Figs. 22–24)

T4b   *Lip and oral cavity:* Tumour invades masticator space, pterygoid plates, or skull base, or encases internal carotid artery (Fig. 25)

Note
Superficial erosion alone of bone/tooth socket by gingival primary is not sufficient to classify a tumour as T4a or T4b

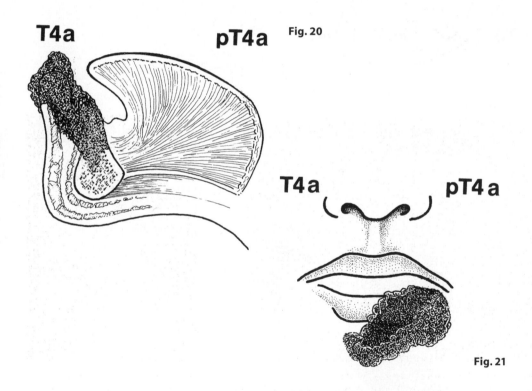

Fig. 20

Fig. 21

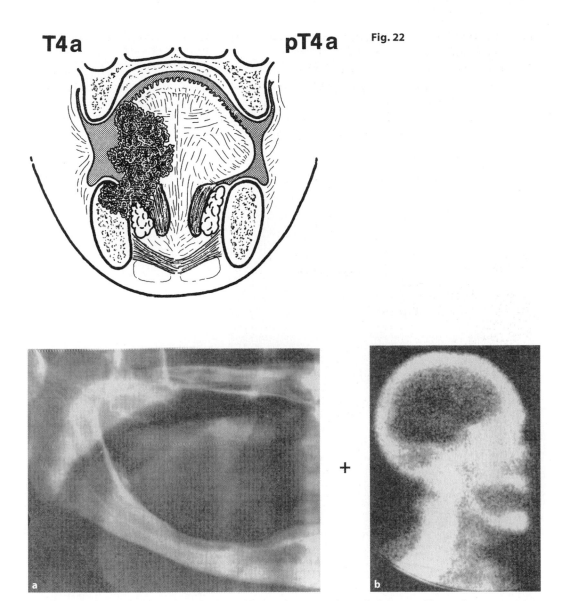

T4a   **pT4a**   Fig. 22

Fig. 23. a Radiographical suspicion but no evidence of invasion through the cortical bone; the tumour must be classified as non-T4a/b in correspondence with the definitions T1, T2 and T3. **b** Evidence of invasion through cortical bone by uptake, which corresponds with the suspected area in the premolar region of the radiograph shown in **a**. On the basis of the scintigraphic finding the tumour must be classified as T4a.

T4a

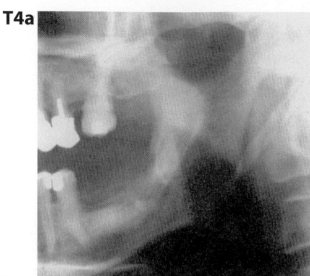

a

T4a

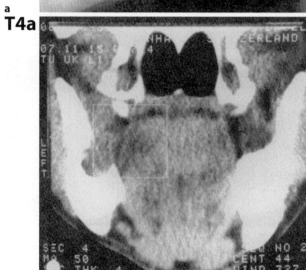

b

Fig. 24. a Evidence of invasion through cortical bone of the mandibula. **b** CT of case shown in **a**. The carcinoma of the floor of the mouth invades through the cortical bone and into the extrinsic muscle of the tongue (m. hyoglossus)

T4b

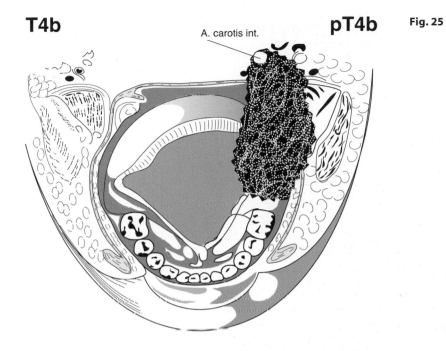

A. carotis int.

pT4b

Fig. 25

N – Regional Lymph Nodes

See p. 6/7.

pTN Pathological Classification

The pT and pN categories correspond to the T and N categories.

Pharynx (ICD-O C01, C05.1, 2, C09, C10.0, 2, 3, C11-13)

Rules for Classification

The classification applies only to carcinomas. There should be histological confirmation of the disease.

Anatomical Sites and Subsites

Oropharynx (C01, C05.1, 2, C09.0, 1, 9, C10.0, 2, 3) (Figs. 26, 27)

1. Anterior wall (glosso-epiglottic area)
   - (i)   Base of tongue (posterior to the vallate papillae or posterior third) (C01)
   - (ii)   Vallecula (C10.0)
2. Lateral wall (C10.2)
   - (i)   Tonsil (C09.9)
   - (ii)   Tonsillar fossa (C09.0) and tonsillar (faucial) pillars (C09.1)
   - (iii) Glossotonsillar sulci (tonsillar pillars) (C09.1)
3. Posterior wall (C10.3)
4. Superior wall
   - (i)   Inferior surface of soft palate (C05.1)
   - (ii)   Uvula (C05.2)

Note
The lingual (anterior) surface of the epiglottis (C10.1) is included with the larynx, suprahyoid epiglottis (see p. 39).

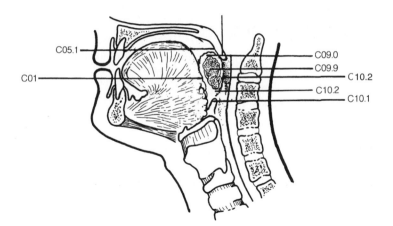

Fig. 26

C05.1
C01
C09.0
C09.9
C10.2
C10.2
C10.1

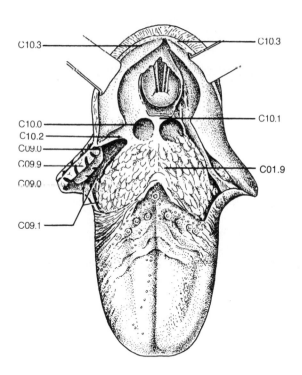

Fig. 27

C10.3
C10.3
C10.0
C10.1
C10.2
C09.0
C09.9
C01.9
C09.0
C09.1

Nasopharynx (C11) (Fig. 28)

1. Postero-superior wall: extends from the level of the junction of the hard and soft palates to the base of the skull (C11.0, 1)
2. Lateral wall: including the fossa of Rosenmüller (C11.2)
3. Inferior wall: consists of the superior surface of the soft palate (C11.3)

Note
The margin of the choanal orifices, including the posterior margin of the nasal septum, is included with the nasal fossa.

Hypopharynx (C12, C13) (Fig. 28)

1. Pharyngo-oesophageal junction (postcricoid area) (C13.0): extends   from the level of the arytenoid cartilages and connecting folds to the inferior border of the cricoid cartilage, thus forming the anterior wall of the hypopharynx.
2. Piriform sinus (C12.9): extends from the pharyngo-epiglottic fold to the upper end of the oesophagus. It is bounded laterally by the thyroid cartilage and medially by the hypopharyngeal surface of the aryepiglottic fold (C13.1) and the arytenoid and cricoid cartilages.
3. Posterior pharyngeal wall (C13.2): extends from the superior level of the hyoid bone (or floor of the vallecula) to the level of the inferior border of the cricoid cartilage and from the apex of one piriform sinus to the other.

Regional Lymph Nodes

The regional lymph nodes are the cervical nodes (see p. 6/7)

The supraclavicular fossa (relevant to classifying nasopharyngeal carcinoma) is the triangular region defined by three points:
(1) the superior margin of the sternal end of the clavicle;
(2) the superior margin of the lateral end of the clavicle;
(3) the point where the neck meets the shoulder:

This includes caudal portions of Levels IV and V (Classification according to Robbins et al.[1])

---

[1] Robbins KT, Median JE, Wolfe GT, Levine PA, Sesions RB, Pruet CW (1991) Standardizing neck dissection terminology. Official report of the Academy's Committee for Head and Neck Surgery and Oncology. Arch Otolaryngol Head Neck Surg 117:601-605

Fig. 28

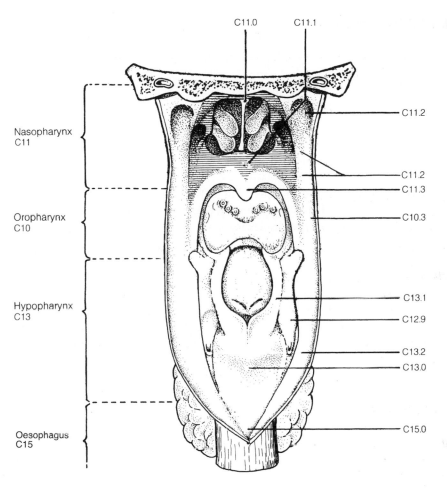

C11.0   C11.1

Nasopharynx
C11

Oropharynx
C10

Hypopharynx
C13

Oesophagus
C15

C11.2

C11.2
C11.3

C10.3

C13.1
C12.9

C13.2
C13.0

C15.0

TN Clinical Classification

T – Primary Tumour

TX   Primary tumour cannot be assessed
T0   No evidence of primary tumour
Tis   Carcinoma in situ

Oropharynx

T1   Tumour 2 cm or less in greatest dimension (Fig. 29)
T2   Tumour more than 2 cm but not more than 4 cm in greatest dimension (Fig. 30)
T3   Tumour more than 4 cm in greatest dimension (Fig. 31)

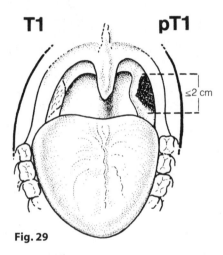

Fig. 29

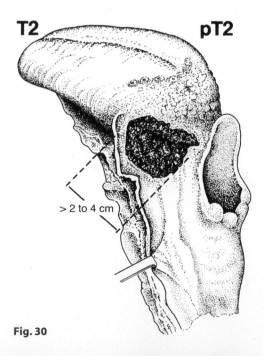

Fig. 30

T3   **pT3**   Fig. 31

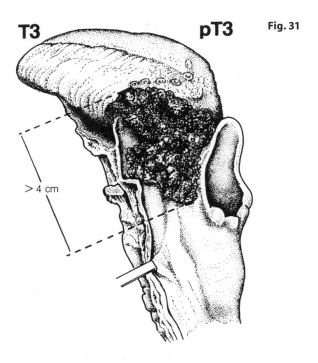

> 4 cm

T4a   Tumour invades any of the following: larynx, deep/extrinsic muscle of tongue (genioglossus, hyoglossus, palatoglossus, and styloglossus), medial pterygoid, hard palate,
and mandible (Fig. 32)

T4a   **pT4a**   Fig. 32

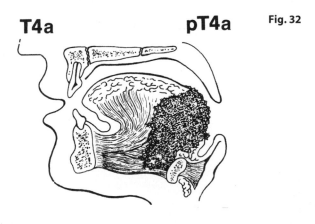

T4b   Tumour invades any of the following: lateral pterygoid muscle, pterygoid plates, lateral nasopharynx, skull base, prevertebral fascia or encases the carotid artery (Fig. 33)

T4b   **pT4b**   **Fig. 33**

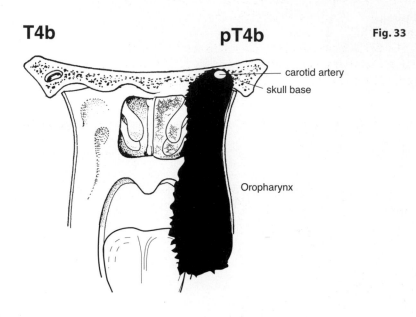

carotid artery
skull base

Oropharynx

Nasopharynx

T1   Tumour confined to nasopharynx (Fig. 34)
T2   Tumour extends to soft tissue of oropharynx and/or nasal cavity (Fig. 34)
    T2a   without parapharyngeal extension* (Fig. 35)
    T2b   with parapharyngeal extension* (Fig. 36)
T3   Tumour invades bony structures and/or paranasal sinuses (Fig. 37)
T4   Tumour with intracranial extension and/or involvement of cranial nerves, infratemporal fossa, hypopharynx, orbit, or masticator space (Fig. 38)

Note
* Parapharyngeal extension denotes postero-lateral infiltration of tumour beyond the pharyngo-basilar fascia.

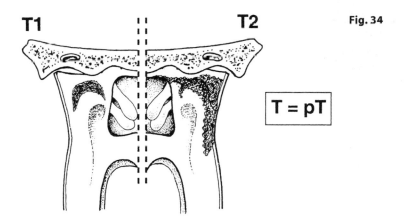

T1   **T2**   **Fig. 34**

$$T = pT$$

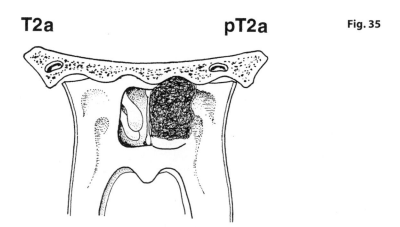

T2a   **pT2a**   **Fig. 35**

T2b   **pT2b**   Fig. 36

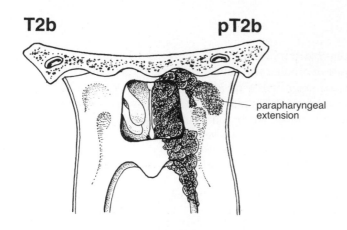

parapharyngeal
extension

T3   **pT3**   Fig. 37

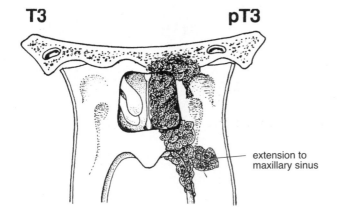

extension to
maxillary sinus

T4   **pT4**   Fig. 38

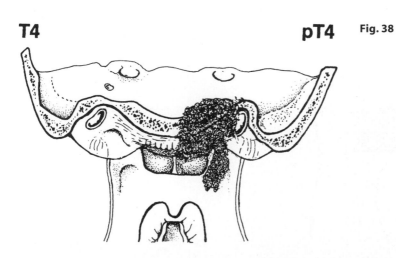

Hypopharynx

T1   Tumour limited to one subsite of hypopharynx (see page 24) and 2 cm or less in greatest dimension (Figs. 39–41)

T2   Tumour invades more than one subsite of hypopharynx or an adjacent site, or measures more than 2 cm but not more than 4 cm in greatest dimension, *without* fixation of hemilarynx (Figs. 42–46)

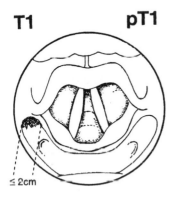

Fig. 39. Involvement of the piriform sinus (C12.9)

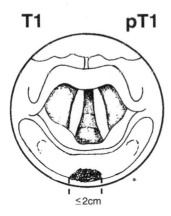

Fig. 40. Involvement of the posterior wall (C13.2)

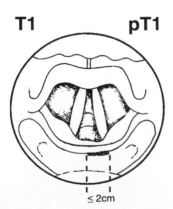

Fig. 41. Involvement of the post-cricoid area (C13.0)

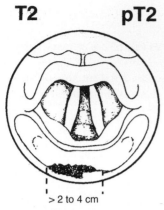

T2   **pT2**

> 2 to 4 cm

Fig. 42. Involvement of the posterior wall of the hypo-pharynx (C13.2)

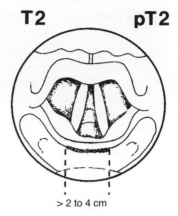

T2   **pT2**

> 2 to 4 cm

Fig. 43. Involvement of the postcricoid area (C13.0)

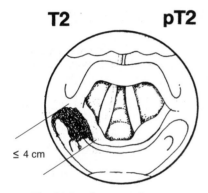

T2   **pT2**

≤ 4 cm

Fig. 44. Involvement of the piriform sinus (C12.9) and the aryepiglottic fold (C13.1)

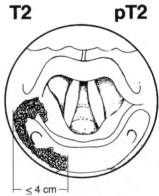

T2   **pT2**

≤ 4 cm

Fig. 45. Involvement of the piriform sinus (C12.9) and the posterior wall of the hypopharynx (C13.2)

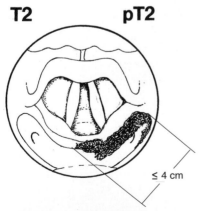

T2   **pT2**

≤ 4 cm

Fig. 46. Involvement of the piriform sinus (C12.9) and the postcricoid area (C13.0)

T3   Tumour measures more than 4 cm in greatest dimension, or with fixation of hemilarynx (Figs. 47–49)

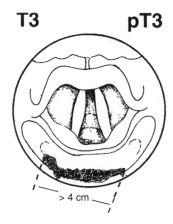

Fig. 47. Involvement of the posterior wall of the hypopharynx (C13.2)

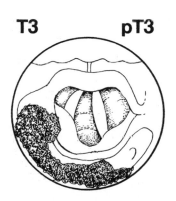

Fig. 48. Invasion of the piriform sinus (C12.9), the aryepiglottic fold (C13.1) and the posterior wall of the hypopharynx (C13.2) with fixation of the hemilarynx

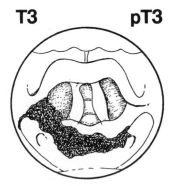

Fig. 49. Invasion of the piriform sinus (C12.9) and postcricoid area (C13.0) with fixation of the hemilarynx

T4a   Tumour invades any of the following: thyroid/cricoid cartilage, hyoid bone, thyroid gland, oesophagus, central compartment soft tissue (Figs. 50–51)

T4b   Tumour invades prevertebral fascia (Fig. 52), encases carotid artery, or invades mediastinal structures

Note
* Central compartment soft tissue includes prelaryngeal strap muscles and subcutaneous fat.

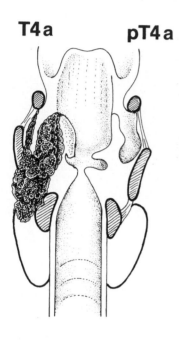

Fig. 50.
Tumors invasion of thyroid cartilage

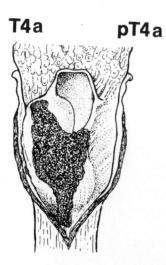

Fig. 51.
Invasion of adjustment oesophagus

T4b

Fig. 52. Tumour invades prevertebral space

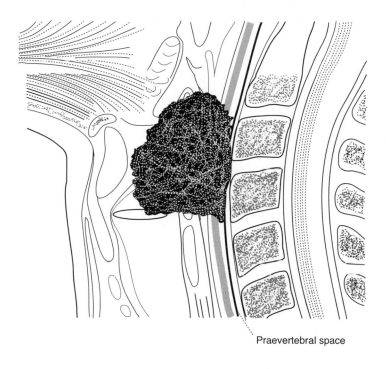

Praevertebral space

Oro- and Hypopharynx

N – Regional Lymph Nodes

See p. 6/7.

Nasopharynx

N – Regional Lymph Nodes

NX   Regional lymph nodes cannot be assessed
N0   No regional lymph node metastasis

N1   Unilateral metastasis in lymph node(s), 6 cm or less in greatest dimension, above su-
       praclavicular fossa (Fig. 53)

Note
Midline nodes are considered ipsilateral nodes.

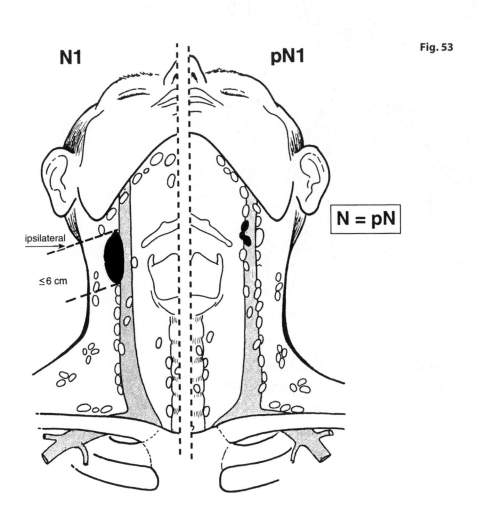

Fig. 53

N2   Bilateral metastasis in lymph node(s), 6 cm or less in greatest dimension, above supra-
     clavicular fossa (Fig. 54)

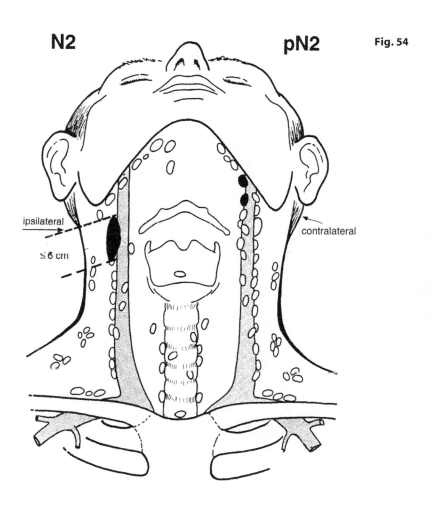

N2   **pN2**   **Fig. 54**

ipsilateral

contralateral

≤ 6 cm

N3   Metastasis in lymph node(s) greater than 6 cm in dimension or in the supraclavicular fossa (Fig. 55)

N3a   greater than 6 cm in dimension
N3b   in the supraclavicular fossa

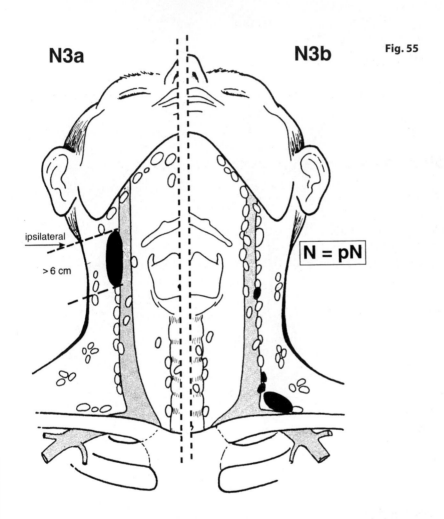

Fig. 55

pTN Pathological Classification

The pT and pN categories correspond to the T and N categories.

Larynx (ICD-O C32.0, 1, 2, C10.1)

Rules for Classification

The classification applies only to carcinomas. There should be histological confirmation of the disease.

Anatomical Sites and Subsites (Figs. 26, 27, p. 23, and Figs. 56, 57)

Supraglottis (C32.1)

(i)   Suprahyoid epiglottis [including tip, lingual (anterior) (C10.1), and laryngeal surfaces]
(ii) Aryepiglottic fold, laryngeal aspect
(iii) Arytenoid

> Epilarynx (including marginal zone)

(iv) Infrahyoid epiglottis
(v)   Ventricular bands (false cords)

> Supraglottis (excluding epilarynx)

Glottis (C32.0)

(i)   Vocal cords
(ii) Anterior commissure
(iii) Posterior commissure

Subglottis (C32.2)

Regional Lymph Nodes

See p. 6/7.

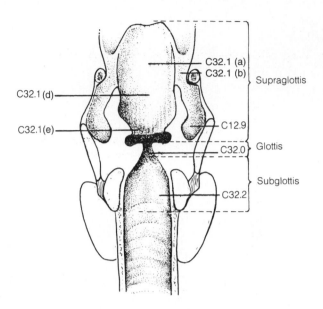

Fig. 56

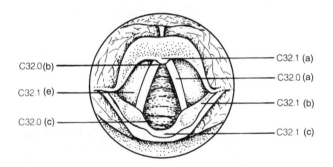

Fig. 57

TN: Clinical Classification

T – Primary Tumour

TX   Primary tumour cannot be assessed
T0   No evidence of primary tumour
Tis   Carcinoma in situ

Supraglottis

T1   Tumour limited to one subsite of supraglottis with normal vocal cord mobility
(Figs. 58a,b, 59a,b)

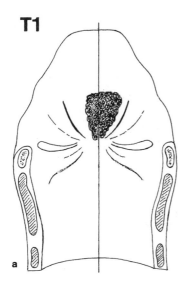
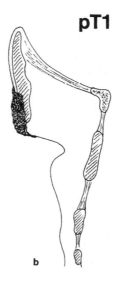

Fig. 58a, b. Involvement of the epiglottis

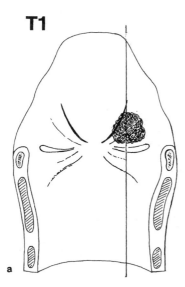
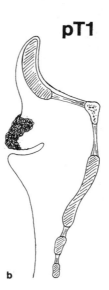

Fig. 59a, b. Involvement of the false cord

Larynx

T2   Tumour invades mucosa of more than one adjacent subsite of supraglottis or glottis or region outside the supraglottis (e.g., mucosa of base of tongue, vallecula, medial wall of piriform sinus) without fixation of the larynx (Figs. 60a,b, 61a,b)

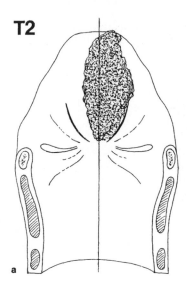

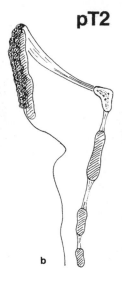

Fig. 60a, b. Involvement of the suprahyoid and the mucosa of the infrahyoid epiglottis

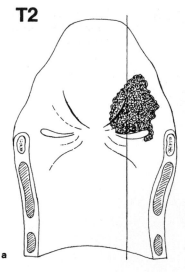

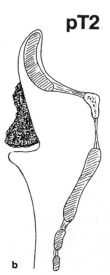

Fig. 61a, b. Involvement of the false cord and the epiglottis

T3   Tumour limited to larynx with vocal cord fixation and/or invades any of the following: postcricoid area, pre-epiglottic tissues, paraglottic space, and/or with minor thyroid cartilage erosion (e.g., inner cortex) (Figs. 62a,b, 63a,b)

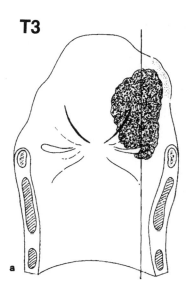

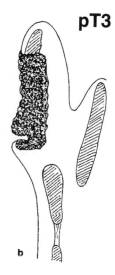

Fig. 62a, b. Involvement of supraglottis and vocal cord with cord fixation

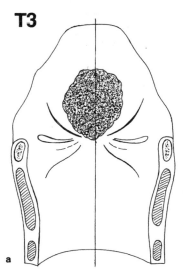

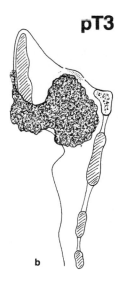

Fig. 63a, b. Invasion of the pre-epiglottic tissues with vocal cord fixation

Larynx

T4a   Tumour invades through thyroid cartilage, and/or invades tissues beyond the lar-
       ynx, e.g., trachea, soft tissues of the neck including deep/extrinsic muscle of tongue
       (genioglossus, hyoglossus, palatoglossus, and styloglossus), strap muscles, thyroid,
       oesophagus (Fig. 64a,b)
T4b   Tumour invades prevertebral space, mediastinal structures, or encases carotid artery
       (Fig. 52)

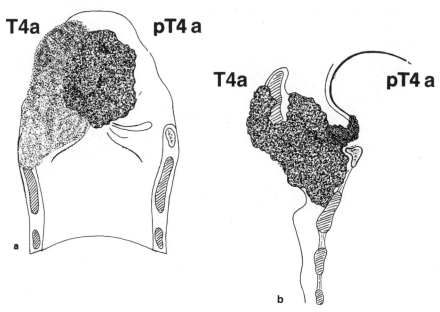

Fig. 64a, b. Invasion beyond the larynx (vallecula and base of tongue) and soft tissues of the neck (pre-
larynx)

Glottis

T1 Tumour limited to vocal cord(s) (may involve anterior or posterior commissure) with normal mobility (Fig. 65a)
    T1a   Tumour limited to one vocal cord (Fig. 65b)
    T1b   Tumour involves both vocal cords (Fig. 65c)
T2 Tumour extends to supraglottis and/or subglottis, and/or with impaired vocal cord mobility (Fig. 66a,b)
T3 Tumour limited to larynx with vocal cord fixation and/or invades paraglottic space, and/or with minor thyroid cartilage erosion (e.g., inner cortex) (Fig. 67a,b)

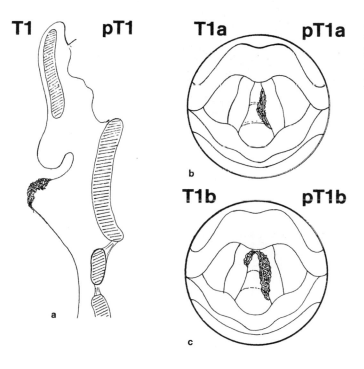

Fig. 65a–c. Tumour limited to vocal cord (**a**, **b**). **c** Tumour limited to vocal cords with invasion of the anterior commissure

Larynx

T2

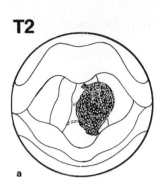

a

pT2

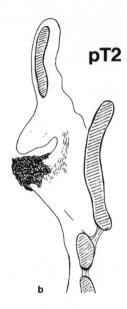

b

Fig. 66a, b. Tumour extends to supraglottis with impaired vocal cord mobility by invasion of the superficial m. vocalis

T3

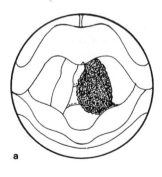

a

pT3

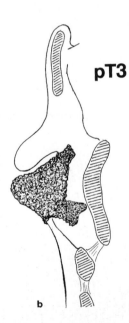

b

Fig. 67a, b. Tumour with vocal cord fixation

T4a   Tumour invades through thyroid cartilage or other tissues beyond the larynx, e.g., trachea, soft tissues of neck including deep/extrinsic muscle of tongue (genioglossus, hyoglossus, palatoglossus, and styloglossus), strap muscles, thyroid, oesophagus (Fig.68a,b)

T4b   Tumour invades prevertebral space, mediastinal structures, or encases carotid artery (Fig. 69)

T4a

pT4a

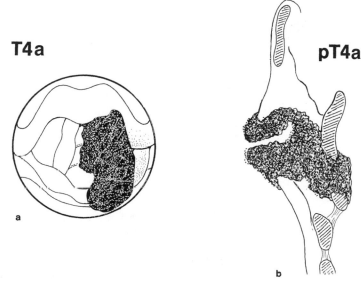

Fig. 68a, b. Tumour invades beyond the larynx (**a**) and invades thyroid cartilage (**b**)

T4b

Fig. 69. Tumour invades prevertebral space

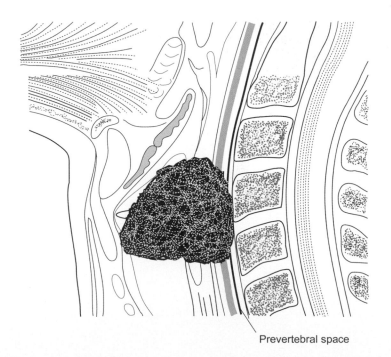

Prevertebral space

Subglottis

T1   Tumour limited to subglottis (Fig. 70)
T2   Tumour extends to vocal cord(s) with normal or impaired mobility (Fig. 71)

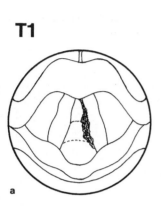

T1

a

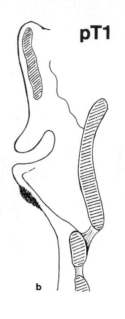

pT1

Fig. 70

b

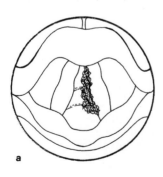

T2

a

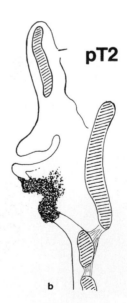

Fig. 71

pT2

b

T3   Tumour limited to larynx with vocal cord fixation (Fig. 72a, b)
T4a   Tumour invades through cricoid or thyroid cartilage and/or invades into other tissues beyond the larynx, e.g., trachea, soft tissues of neck including deep/extrinsic muscle of tongue (genioglossus, hyoglossus, palatoglossus, and styloglossus), strap muscles, thyroid, oesophagus (Fig. 73a, b)

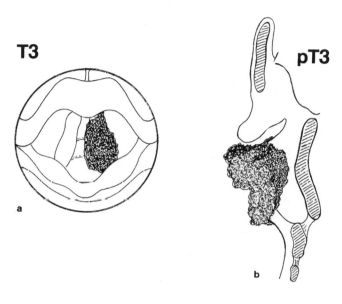

Fig. 72a, b. Tumour with vocal cord fixation

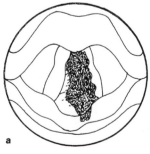
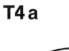
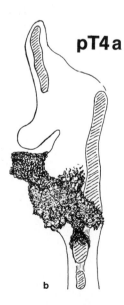

Fig. 73a, b. Tumour invades through thyroid cartilage

Larynx

T4b   Tumour invades prevertebral space, mediastinal structures, or encases carotid artery (Fig. 74)

T4b

Fig. 74. Tumour invades prevertebral space

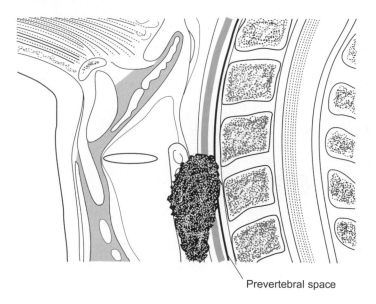

Prevertebral space

N – Regional Lymph Nodes

See p. 6/7.

pTN Pathological Classification

The pT and pN categories correspond to the T and N categories.

Nasal Cavity and Paranasal Sinuses

(ICD-O C30.0, C31.0,1)

Rules for Classification

The classification applies only to carcinomas. There should be histological confirmation of the disease.

Anatomical Sites and Subsites

1. **Nasal Cavity** *(C30.0)* (Fig. 75)
   – Septum
   – Floor
   – Lateral wall
   – Vestibule
2. **Maxillary sinus** *(C31.0)* (Fig. 76)
3. **Ethmoid sinus** *(C31.1)* (Fig. 76)
   – Left
   – Right

Regional Lymph Nodes

See p. 6/7.

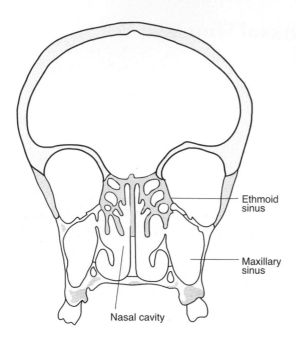

Fig. 75

Ethmoid
sinus

Maxillary
sinus

Nasal cavity

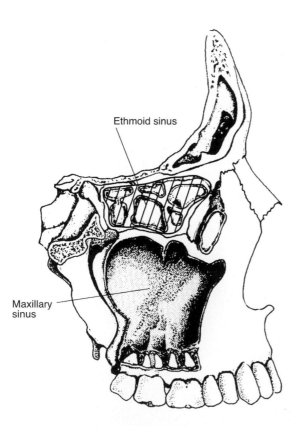

Fig. 76

Ethmoid sinus

Maxillary
sinus

TN Clinical Classification

T – Primary Tumour

TX   Primary tumour cannot be assessed
T0   No evidence of primary tumour
Tis   Carcinoma in situ

Maxillary Sinus

T1   Tumour limited to the antral mucosa with no erosion or destruction of bone (Fig. 77)
T2   Tumour causing bone erosion or destruction including extension into hard palate and/or middle nasal meatus, except extension to posterior wall of maxillary sinus and pterygoid plates (Fig. 78)

T1   **pT1**   **Fig. 77**

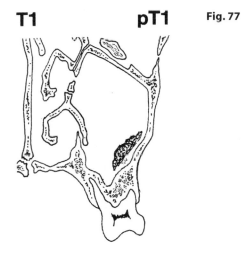

T2   **pT2**   **Fig. 78**

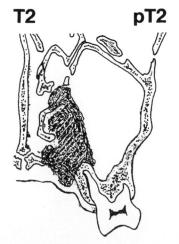

T3   Tumour invades any of the following: bone of posterior wall of maxillary sinus, subcutaneous tissues, floor or medial wall of orbit, ptergoid fossa, ethmoid sinuses (Figs. 79, 80)

T3   **T3**

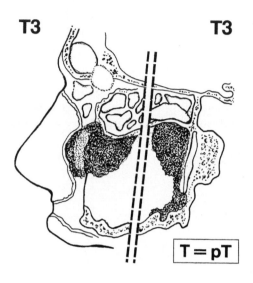

Fig. 79

T3   **T3**

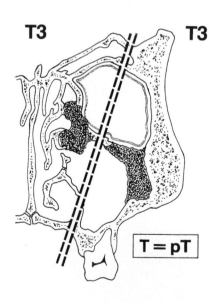

Fig. 80 Tumor of the maxillary sinus with invasion of the medial wall of the orbit and of ethmoid sinus

T4a   Tumour invades any of the following: anterior orbital contents, skin of cheeck, ptery-
       goid plates, infratemporal fossa, cribriform plate, sphenoid or frontal sinuses (Figs. 81,
       82)

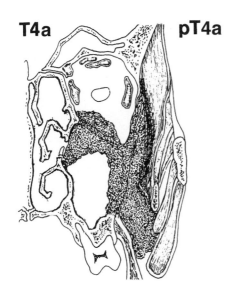

T4a   **pT4a**

Fig. 81

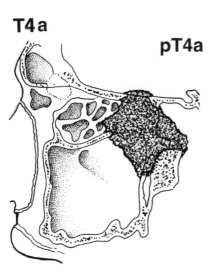

T4 a

pT4a

Fig. 82

T4b   Tumour invades any of the following: orbital apex, dura, brain, middle cranial fossa, cranial nerves other than maxillary division of trigeminal nerve (V2), nasopharynx, clivus (Fig. 83)

T4b   **pT4b**   Fig. 83

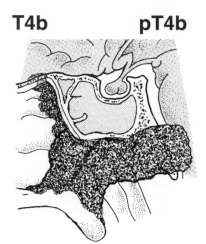

Nasal Cavity and Ethmoid Sinus

T1   Tumour restricted to one subsite of nasal cavity or ethmoid sinus, with or without bony invasion (Figs. 84, 85)

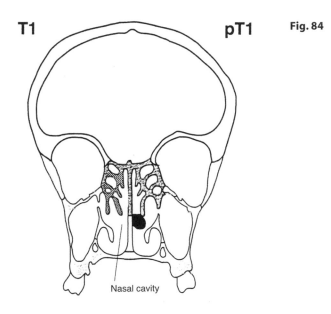

T1   **pT1**   **Fig. 84**

Nasal cavity

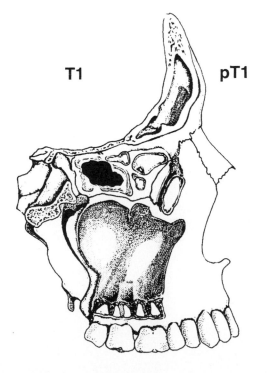

Fig. 85

T1   **pT1**

T2   Tumour involves two subsites in a single site or extends to involve an adjacent site within the nasoethmoidal complex, with or without bony invasion (Fig. 86)

T3   Tumour extends to invade the medial wall or floor of the orbit, maxillary sinus, palate, or cribriform plate (Fig. 87)

T2   **pT2**

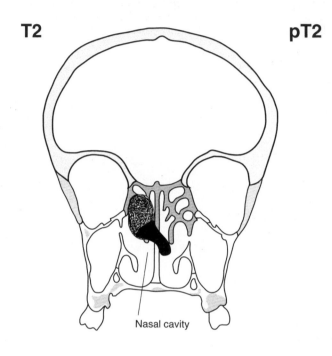

Nasal cavity

Fig. 86. Tumour of ethmoid with extension to nasal cavity

T3   **T3**

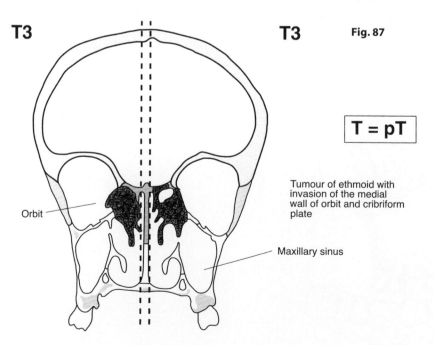

Orbit

Maxillary sinus

Fig. 87

T = pT

Tumour of ethmoid with invasion of the medial wall of orbit and cribriform plate

T4a   Tumour invades any of the following: anterior orbital contents, skin of nose or cheeck, minimal extension to anterior cranial fossa, pterygoid plates, sphenoid or frontal sinuses (Fig. 88)

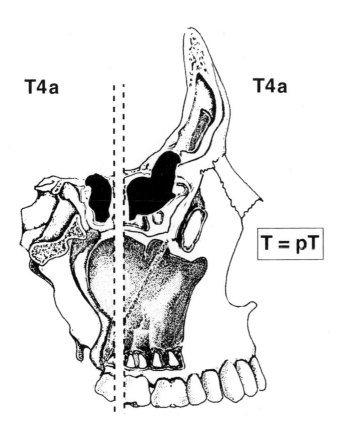

T4a   **T4a**

T = pT

Fig. 88. Tumor of ethmoid sinus with invasion of frontal sinuses and anterior cranial fossa

T4b   Tumour invades any of the following: orbital apex, dura, brain, middle cranial fossa, cranial nerves other than V2, nasopharynx, clivus (Fig. 89)

Fig. 89

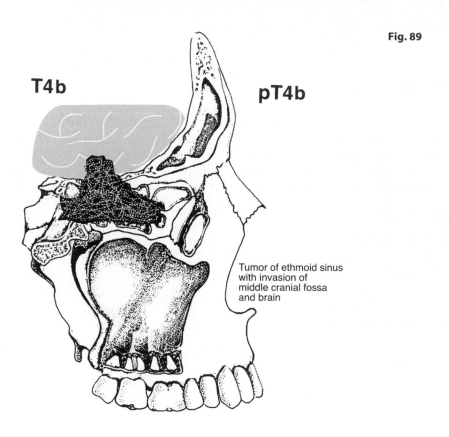

T4b   pT4b

Tumor of ethmoid sinus
with invasion of
middle cranial fossa
and brain

N – Regional Lymph Nodes

See p. 6/7.

pTN Pathological Classification

The pT and pN classification correspond to the T and N categories.

Salivary Glands (ICD-O C07, C08)

Rules for Classification

The classification applies only to carcinomas of the major salivary glands: parotid (C07.9), submandibular (submaxillary) (C08.0), and sublingual (C08.1) glands. Tumours arising in minor salivary glands (mucus-secreting glands in the lining membrane of the upper aerodigestive tract) are not included in this classification but at their anatomic site of origin, e.g., lip. There should be histological confirmation of the disease.

Regional Lymph Nodes

The regional lymph nodes are the cervical nodes (see page 6/7).

TNM Clinical Classification

T – Primary Tumour

TX   Primary tumour cannot be assessed
T0   No evidence of primary tumour

T1   Tumour 2 cm or less in greatest dimension without extraparenchymal extension* (Fig. 90)
T2   Tumour more than 2 cm but not more than 4 cm in greatest dimension without extraparenchymal extension* (Fig. 91)

Note
* Extraparenchymal extension is clinical or macroscopic evidence of invasion of soft tissues or nerve, except these listed under T4a and T4b. Microscopic evidence alone does not constitute extraparenchymal extension for classification purposes.

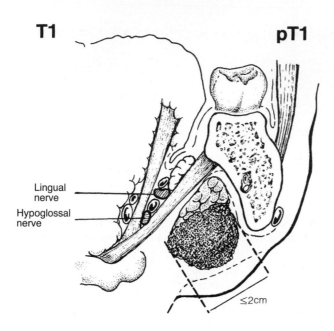

T1   **pT1**

Lingual
nerve
Hypoglossal
nerve

≤2cm

Fig. 90. Classification determined clinically on the basis of absence of paralysis or macroscopically on the basis of no extraparenchymal extension. Frontal section through the premolar region

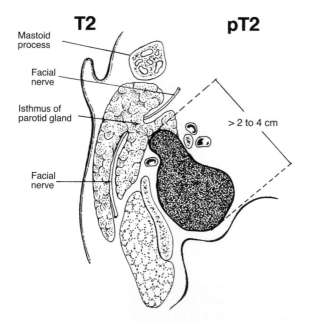

T2   **pT2**

Mastoid
process
Facial
nerve
Isthmus of
parotid gland

> 2 to 4 cm

Facial
nerve

Fig. 91. Horizontal section through the parotid gland showing its supposed division into superficial and deep lobes

T3 Tumour more than 4 cm and/or tumour having extraparenchymal extension* (Figs. 92, 93)

Note
See p. 61.

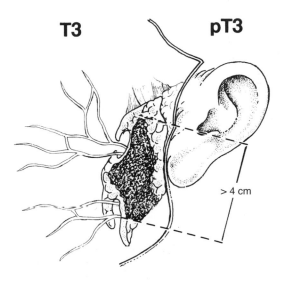

Fig. 92
Tumour more than 4 cm without extraparenchymal extension

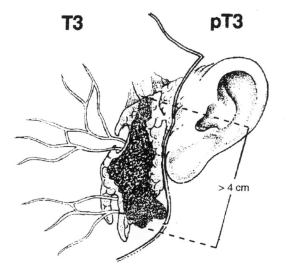

Fig. 93
Tumour more than 4 cm with extraparenchymal extension

▌T4a   Tumour invades skin, mandible, ear canal, or facial nerve (Fig. 94)

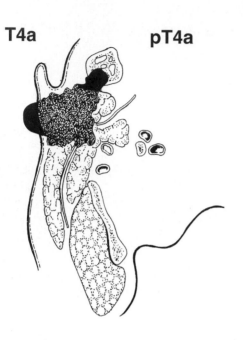

Fig. 94. Invasion of the facial nerve and of skin

▎T4b   Tumour invades base of skull, pterygoid plates, or encases carotid artery (Fig. 95)

pT4b

Fig. 95

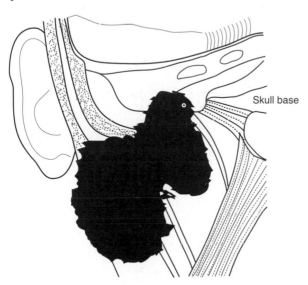

Skull base

N – Regional Lymph Nodes

See p. 6/7.

pTN Pathological Classification

The pT and pN categories correspond to the T and N categories.

Thyroid Gland (ICD-O C73) (Fig. 96)

Rules for Classification

The classification applies only to carcinomas. There should be microscopic confirmation of the disease and division of cases by histological type.

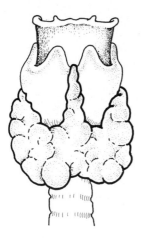

Fig. 96

Regional Lymph Nodes (Fig. 97)

The regional lymph nodes are the cervical and upper/superior mediastinal nodes.

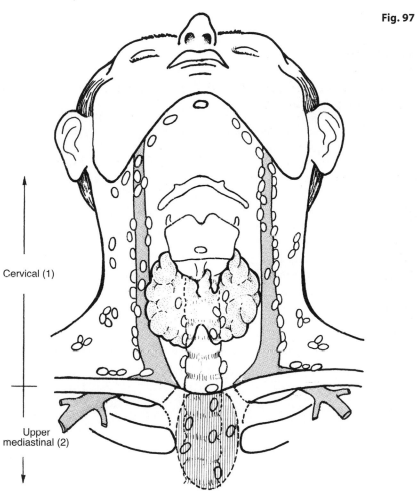

Fig. 97

Cervical (1)

Upper
mediastinal (2)

TN Clinical Classification

T – Primary Tumour

TX   Primary tumour cannot be assessed
T0   No evidence of primary tumour

All instological types except undifferentiated carcinoma
T1   Tumour 2 cm or less in greatest dimension, limited to the thyroid (Fig. 98)
T2   Tumour more than 2 cm but not more than 4 cm in greatest dimension, limited to the thyroid (Fig. 99)
T3   Tumour more than 4 cm in greatest dimension, limited to the thyroid or any tumour with minimal extrathyroidal extension (e.g., extension to sternothyroid muscle or perithyroid soft tissues) (Figs. 100, 101)
T4a   Tumour extends beyond the thyroid capsule and invades any of the following: subcutaneous soft tissues, larynx, trachea, oesophagus, recurrent laryngeal nerve (Fig. 102)
T4b   Tumour invades prevertebral fascia, mediastinal vessels or encases carotid artery (Fig. 103)

Undifferentiated carcinoma (all are classified as T4)
T4a   Tumour (any size) limited to the thyroid, considered surgically resectable
T4b   Tumour (any size) extends beyond the thyroid capsule, considered surgically unresectable

Note
Multifocal tumours should be designated (m) (the largest determines the classification), e.g., T2(m).

T1 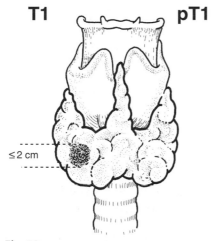 **pT1**

≤ 2 cm

Fig. 98

T2 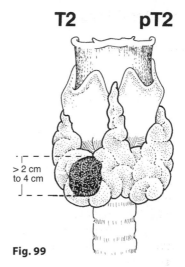 **pT2**

> 2 cm to 4 cm

Fig. 99

T3 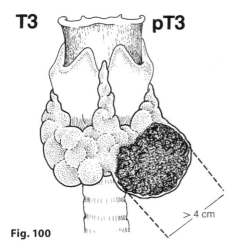 **pT3**

> 4 cm

Fig. 100

T3 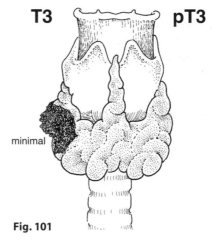 **pT3**

minimal

Fig. 101

Thyroid Gland

T4a   pT4a   Fig. 102

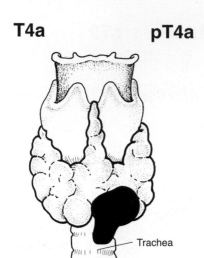

Trachea

T4b   pT4b   Fig. 103

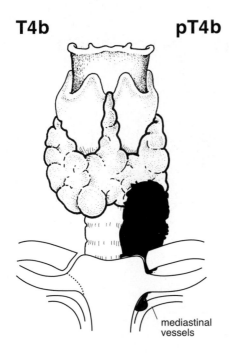

mediastinal
vessels

N – Regional Lymph Nodes

NX   Regional lymph nodes cannot be assessed
N0   No regional lymph node metastasis
N1a   Metastasis in Level VI (pretracheal, paratracheal, including prelaryngeal and Delphian lymph node(s)) (see p. 6) (Fig. 104)
N1b   Metastasis in other unilateral, bilateral, or contralateral cervical or upper/superior mediastinal lymph node(s) (Fig. 105)

pTNM Pathological Classification

The pT, pN, and pM categories correspond to the T, N, and M categories.

pN0 Histological examination of a selective neck dissection specimen will ordinarily include 6 or more lymph nodes.
    If the examined lymph nodes are negative, but the number ordinarily resected is not met, classify as pN0.

N1a   **pN1a**   **Fig. 104**

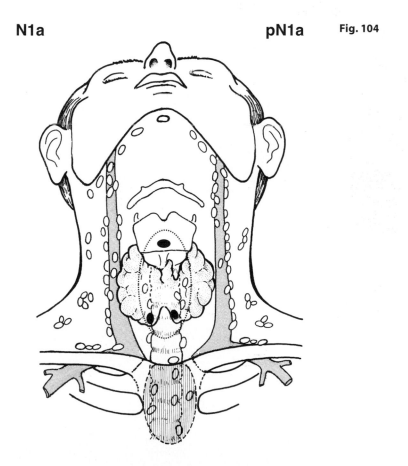

Thyroid Gland

N1b   **pN1b**   Fig. 105

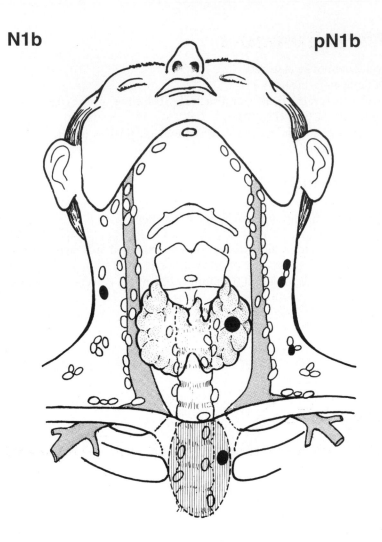

Digestive System Tumours

Introductory Notes

The following sites are included:

- Oesophagus
- Stomach
- Small Intestine
- Colon and Rectum
- Anal Canal
- Liver
- Gallbladder
- Extrahepatic Bile Ducts
- Ampulla of Vater
- Pancreas

Regional Lymph Nodes

The number of lymph nodes ordinarily included in a lymphadenectomy specimen is noted at each site.

Oesophagus (ICD-O C15)

Rules for Classification

The classification applies only to carcinomas. There should be histological confirmation of the disease and division of cases by histological type.

Anatomical Subsites (Fig. 106)

1. **Cervical oesophagus** (C15.0):
    This commences at the lower border of the cricoid cartilage and ends at the thoracic inlet (suprasternal notch), approximately 18 cm from the upper incisor teeth.
2. **Intrathoracic oesophagus**
    (i)   The upper thoracic portion (C15.3) extending from the thoracic inlet to the level of the tracheal bifurcation, approximately 24 cm from the upper incisor teeth.
    (ii) The mid-thoracic portion (C15.4) is the proximal half of the oesophagus between the tracheal bifurcation and the oesophagogastric junction. The lower level is approximately 32 cm from the upper incisor teeth.
    (iii) The lower thoracic portion (C15.5), approximately 8 cm in length (includes abdominal oesophagus), is the distal half of the oesophagus between the tracheal bifurcation and the oesophagogastric junction. The lower level is approximately 40 cm from the upper incisor teeth.

Fig. 106

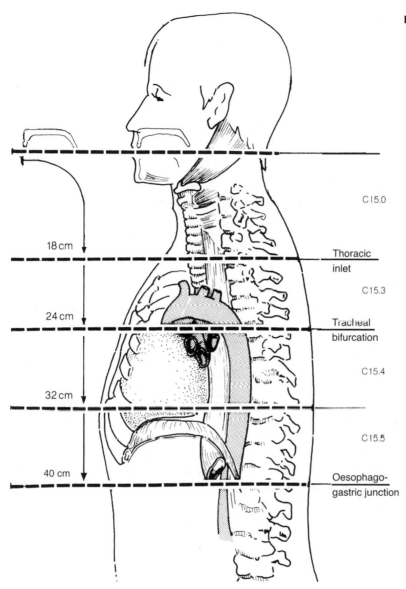

18 cm

24 cm

32 cm

40 cm

C 15.0

Thoracic
inlet

C15.3

Tracheal
bifurcation

C15.4

C 15.5

Oesophago-
gastric junction

Regional Lymph Nodes

The regional lymph nodes are as follows (Fig. 107):

Cervical oesophagus:
- Scalene
- Internal jugular
- Upper and lower cervical
- Perioesophageal
- Supraclavicular

Intrathoracic oesophagus – upper, middle, and lower:
- Upper perioesophgeal (above the azygos vein)
- Subcarinal
- Lower perioesophageal (below the azygos vein)
- Mediastinal lymph nodes
- Perigastric lymph nodes (except coeliac lymph nodes)

Fig. 107

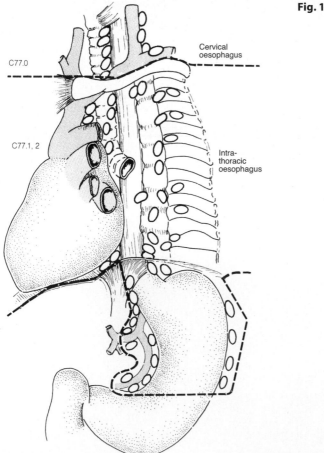

C77.0

C77.1, 2

Cervical
oesophagus

Intra-
thoracic
oesophagus

TNM Clinical Classification

T – Primary Tumour

TX   Primary tumour cannot be assessed
T0   No evidence of primary tumour
Tis   Carcinoma in situ

T1   Tumour invades lamina propria or submucosa (Fig. 108)
T2   Tumour invades muscularis propria (Fig. 109)

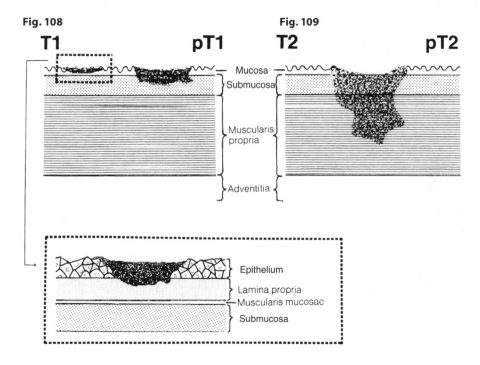

Fig. 108

Fig. 109

T3   Tumour invades adventitia (Fig. 110)
T4   Tumour invades adjacent structures (Fig. 111)

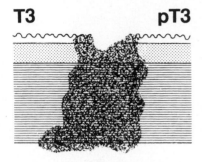

Fig. 110

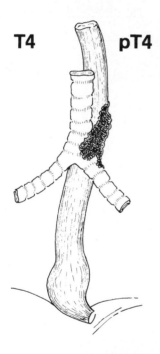

Fig. 111

N – Regional Lymph Nodes

NX   Regional lymph nodes cannot be assessed
N0   No regional lymph node metastasis
N1   Regional lymph node metastasis (Figs. 112–115)

Fig. 112

Carcinoma of cervical oesophagus

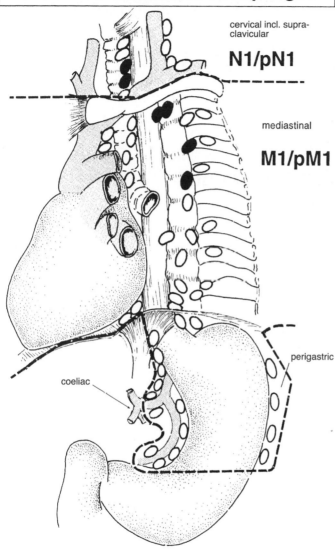

cervical incl. supra-clavicular

N1/pN1

mediastinal

M1/pM1

perigastric

coeliac

Fig. 113

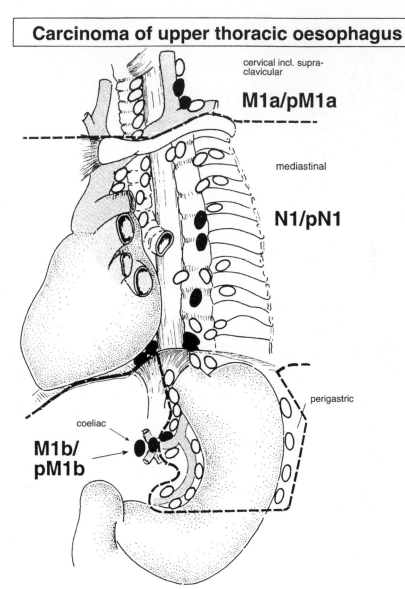

Carcinoma of upper thoracic oesophagus

cervical incl. supra-clavicular

M1a/pM1a

mediastinal

N1/pN1

perigastric

coeliac

M1b/ pM1b

Fig. 114

Carcinoma of mid-thoracic oesophagus

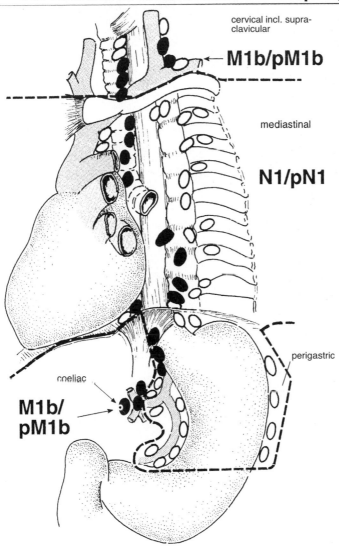

cervical incl. supra-
clavicular

M1b/pM1b

mediastinal

N1/pN1

perigastric

coeliac

M1b/
pM1b

Carcinoma of lower thoracic oesophagus

Fig. 115

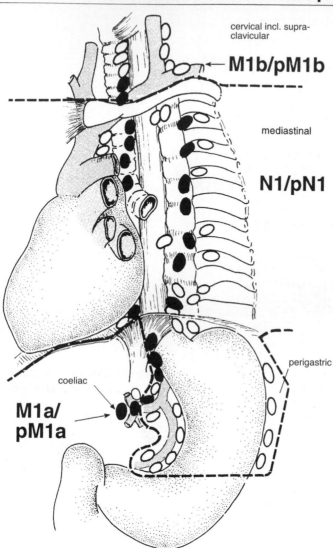

cervical incl. supra-
clavicular

M1b/pM1b

mediastinal

N1/pN1

perigastric

coeliac

M1a/
pM1a

M – Distant Metastasis

MX   Distant metastasis cannot be assessed
M0   No distant metastasis
M1   Distant metastasis

For tumours of lower thoracic oesophagus (Fig. 115)
M1a   Metastasis in coeliac lymph nodes
M1b   Other distant metastasis

For tumours of upper thoracic oesophagus (Fig. 113)
M1a   Metastasis in cervical lymph nodes
M1b   Other distant metastasis

For tumours of mid-thoracic oesophagus (Fig. 114)
M1a   Not applicable
M1b   Non-regional lymph nodes or other distant metastasis

pTN Pathological Classification

The pT, pN, and pM categories correspond to the T, N, and M categories.

pN0 Histological examination of a mediastinal lymphadenectomy specimen will ordinarily include 6 or more lymph nodes. If the examined lymph nodes are negative, but the number ordinarily resected is not met, classify as pN0.

Stomach (ICD-O C16)

Rules for Classification

The classification applies only to carcinomas. There should be histological confirmation of the disease.

Anatomical Subsites (Fig. 116)

1. Cardia (gastroesophageal junction) (C16.0)
2. Fundus (C16.1)
3. Corpus (C16.2)
4. Antrum (C16.3) and pylorus (C16.4)

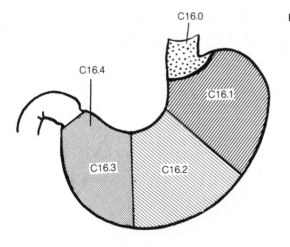

Fig. 116

Regional Lymph Nodes (Figs. 117, 118)

The regional lymph nodes of the stomach are the perigastric nodes along the lesser (1, 3, 5) and greater curvatures(2, 4a, 4b), the nodes along the left gastric (7), common hepatic (8), splenic (11), and coeliac arteries (9), and the hepatoduodenal nodes (12).

The regional lymph nodes of the gastroesophageal junction are the paracardial (1, 2), left gastric (7), coeliac (9), diaphragmatic, and the lower mediastinal paraoesophageal (see p. 76, Fig. 107).

Involvement of other intra-abdominal lymph nodes such as retropancreatic, mesenteric, and para-aortic is classified as distant metastasis.

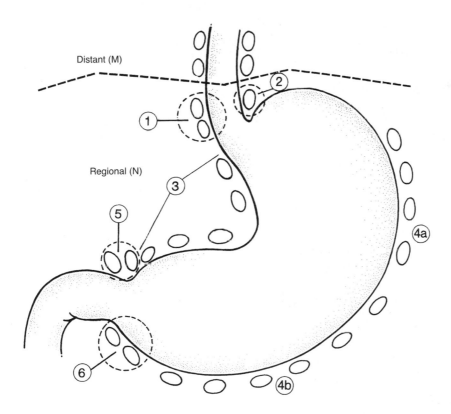

Fig. 117

Note

The numerical order corresponds to the proposals of the Japanese Gastric Cancer Society (1998) Japanese Classification of Gastric Carcinoma, 2nd English edition. Gastric Cancer 1:10–24

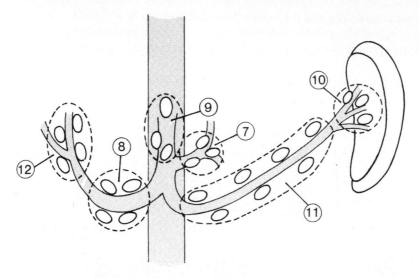

Fig. 118 Regional lymph nodes of the stomach

TNM Clinical Classification

T – Primary Tumour

TX   Primary tumour cannot be assessed
T0   No evidence of primary tumour
Tis   Carcinoma in situ: intraepithelial tumour without invasion of the lamina propria

T1   Tumour invades lamina propria or submucosa (Fig. 119)
T2   Tumour invades muscularis propria or subserosa
    T2a   Tumour invades muscularis propria (Fig. 119)
    T2b   Tumour invades subserosa (Figs. 119–121)

Note
See p. 89.

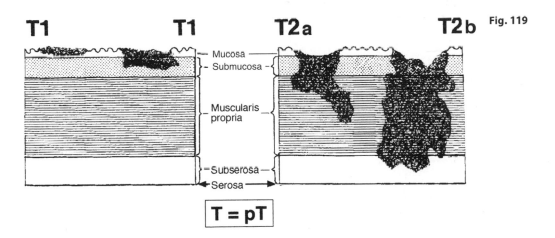

Fig. 119

$T = pT$

T2b

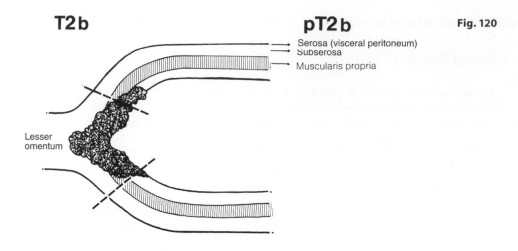

pT2b   Fig. 120

→ Serosa (visceral peritoneum)
→ Subserosa
→ Muscularis propria

Lesser
omentum

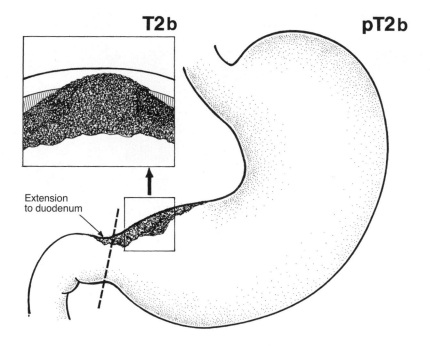

T2b   pT2b   Fig. 121

Extension
to duodenum

T3   Tumour penetrates serosa (visceral peritoneum) without invasion of adjacent structures[1,2,3] (Figs. 122–124)

T4   Tumour invades adjacent structures[1,2,3] (Fig. 122)

Notes

[1] A tumour may penetrate muscularis propria with extension into the gastrocolic or gastrohepatic ligaments or the greater and lesser omentum without perforation of the visceral peritoneum covering these structures. In this case, the tumour is classified as T2b. If there is perforation of the visceral peritoneum covering the gastric ligaments or omenta, the tumour is classified as T3 (Fig. 123).

[2] The adjacent structures of the stomach are the spleen, transverse colon, liver, diaphragm, pancreas, abdominal wall, adrenal gland, kidney, small intestine, and retroperitoneum.

[3] Intramural extension to the duodenum or oesophagus is classified by the depth of greatest invasion in any of these sites including stomach (Figs. 121, 124).

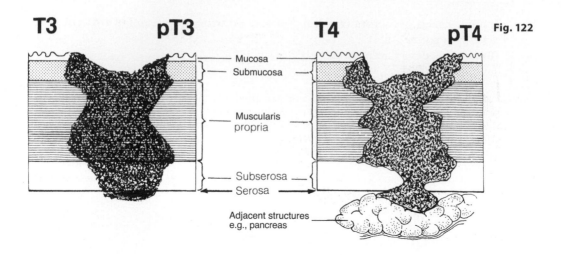

T3 **pT3** **T4** **pT4** **Fig. 122**

Mucosa
Submucosa
Muscularis propria
Subserosa
Serosa
Adjacent structures e.g., pancreas

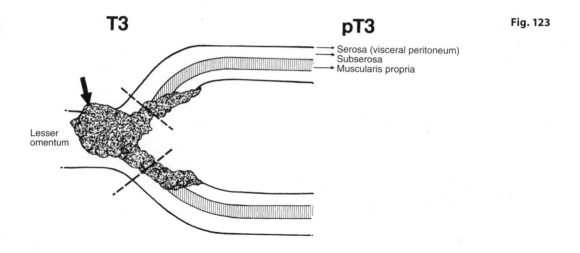

T3 **pT3** **Fig. 123**

Serosa (visceral peritoneum)
Subserosa
Muscularis propria

Lesser omentum

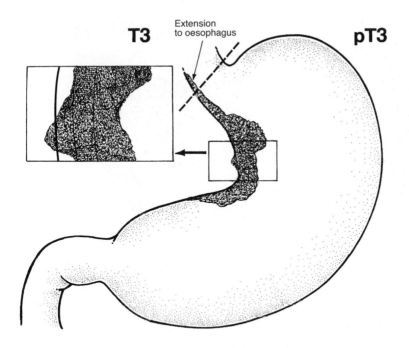

Fig. 124

N – Regional Lymph Nodes

NX   Regional lymph nodes cannot be assessed
N0   No regional lymph node metastasis
N1   Metastasis in 1 to 6 regional lymph nodes (Fig. 125)
N2   Metastasis in 7 to 15 regional lymph nodes (Fig. 126)
N3   Metastasis in more than 15 regional lymph nodes (Fig. 127)

N1

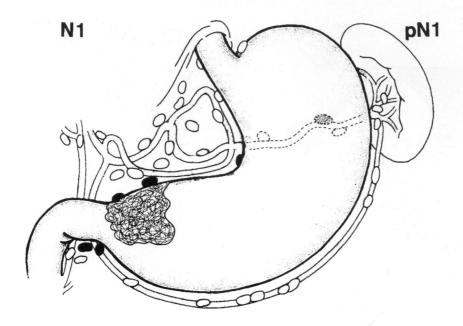

pN1

Fig. 125

N2

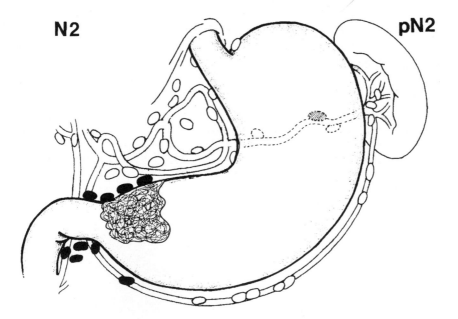

pN2

Fig. 126

N3

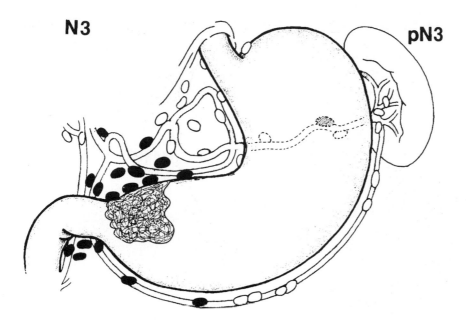

pN3

Fig. 127

M – Distant Metastasis

MX   Distant metastasis cannot be assessed
M0   No distant metastasis
M1   Distant metastasis (Fig. 128)

M1   **pM1**   **Fig. 128**

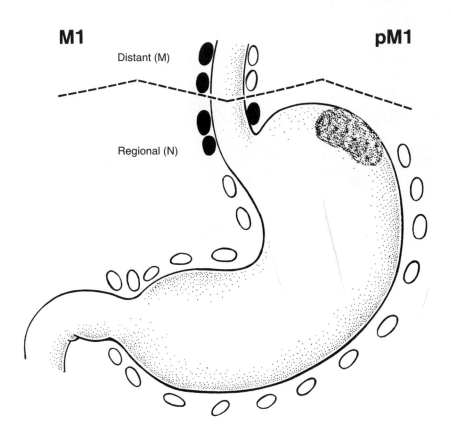

Distant (M)

Regional (N)

pTNM Pathological Classification

The pT, pN, and pM categories correspond to the T, N, and M categories.

pN0 Histological examination of a regional lymphadenectomy specimen will ordinarily include more than 15 lymph nodes. If the examined lymph nodes are negative, but the number ordinarily resected is not met, classify as pN0.

Small Intestine (ICD-O C17)

Rules for Classification

The classification applies only to carcinomas. There should be histological confirmation of the disease.

Anatomical Subsites (Fig. 129)

1. Duodenum (C17.0)
2. Jejunum (C17.1)
3 Ileum (C17.2) (excludes ileocaecal valve C18.0)

Note
This classification does not apply to carcinomas of the ampulla of Vater (see p. 140ff.).

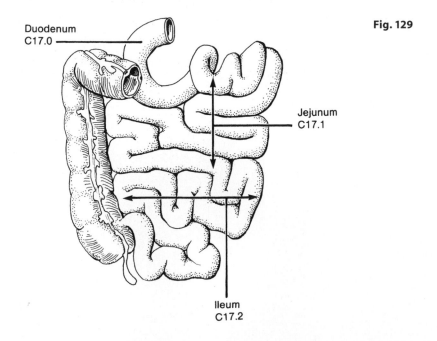

Duodenum
C17.0

Fig. 129

Jejunum
C17.1

Ileum
C17.2

Regional Lymph Nodes

The regional lymph nodes for the duodenum are the pancreaticoduodenal, pyloric, hepatic (pericholedochal, cystic, hilar), and superior mesenteric nodes.

The regional lymph nodes for the ileum and jejunum are the mesenteric nodes, including the superior mesenteric nodes, and, for the terminal ileum only, the ileocolic nodes including the posterior cecal nodes.

TNM Clinical Classification

T – Primary Tumour

TX   Primary tumour cannot be assessed
T0   No evidence of primary tumour
Tis   Carcinoma in situ

T1   Tumour invades lamina propria or submucosa (Fig. 130)
T2   Tumour invades muscularis propria (Fig. 131)
T3   Tumour invades through muscularis propria into subserosa or into non-peritoneal-ized perimuscular tissue (mesentery or retroperitoneum*) with extension 2 cm or less (Figs. 132, 134)
T4   Tumour perforates visceral peritoneum or directly invades other organs or structures (includes other loops of small intestine, mesentery, or retroperitoneum more than 2 cm and abdominal wall by way of serosa; for duodenum only, invasion of pancreas) (Figs. 133–136)

Note
* The non-peritonealized perimuscular tissue is, for jejunum and ileum, part of the mesentery and, for duodenum in areas where serosa is lacking, part of the retroperitoneum (Fig. 134).

Small Intestine

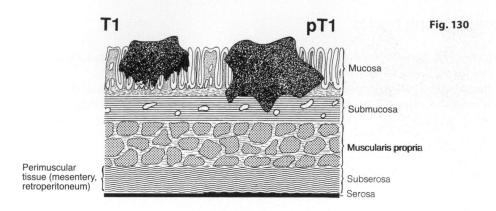

T1   **pT1**   Fig. 130

Mucosa

Submucosa

Muscularis propria

Perimuscular
tissue (mesentery,
retroperitoneum)

Subserosa

Serosa

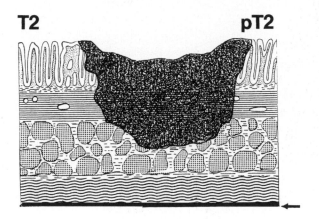

T2   **pT2**   Fig. 131

T3

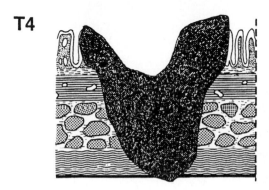

Subserosa
Serosa

Fig. 132

T4

Fig. 133

T3   **T4**   Fig. 134

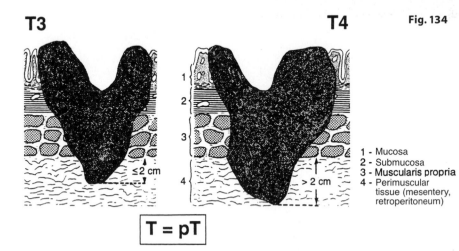

1 - Mucosa
2 - Submucosa
3 - **Muscularis propria**
4 - Perimuscular
tissue (mesentery,
retroperitoneum)

≤ 2 cm
> 2 cm

$$T = pT$$

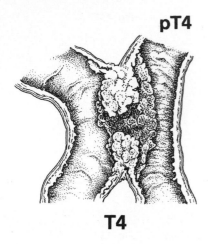

pT4

Fig. 135

T4

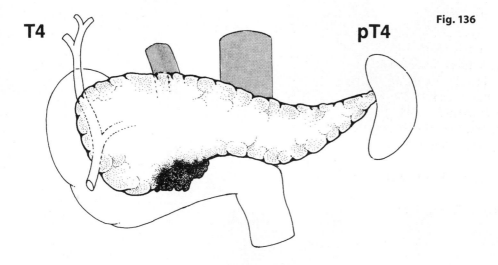

T4

pT4

Fig. 136

N – Regional Lymph Nodes

NX   Regional lymph nodes cannot be assessed
N0   No regional lymph node metastasis
N1   Regional lymph node metastasis

pTN Pathological Classification

The pT and pN categories correspond to the T and N categories.

pN0 Histological examination of a regional lymphadenectomy specimen will ordinarily include 6 or more lymph nodes. If the examined lymph nodes are negative, but the number ordinarily resected is not met, classify as pN0.

Colon and Rectum (ICD-O C18-C20)

Rules for Classification

The classification applies only to carcinomas. There should be histological confirmation of the disease.

Anatomical Subsites

Colon (C18) (Fig. 137)
1. Appendix (18.1)
2. Caecum (C18.0)
3. Ascending colon (C18.2)
4. Hepatic flexure (C18.3)
5. Transverse colon (C18.4)
6. Splenic flexure (C18.5)
7. Descending colon (C18.6)
8. Sigmoid colon (C18.7)

Rectosigmoid Junction (C19) (Fig. 138)

Rectum (C20) (Fig. 138)

Fig. 137

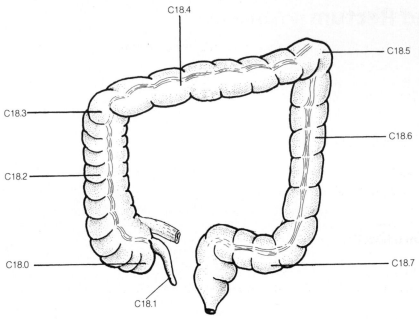
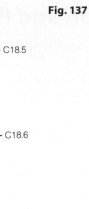

C18.4

C18.5

C18.3

C18.6

C18.2

C18.0

C18.7

C18.1

Fig. 138

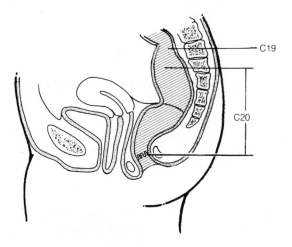

C19

C20

Regional Lymph Nodes

For each anatomical subsite the following are the regional lymph nodes:

Appendix (Fig. 139)
> ileocolic lymph nodes

Caecum (Fig. 140)
> ileocolic, right colic lymph nodes

Ascending colon (Fig. 141)
> ileocolic, right colic, middle colic lymph nodes

Hepatic flexure (Fig. 142)
> right colic, middle colic lymph nodes

Transverse colon (Fig. 143)
> right colic, middle colic, left colic, inferior mesenteric lymph nodes

Splenic flexure (Fig. 144)
> middle colic, left colic, inferior mesenteric lymph nodes

Descending colon (Fig.145)
> left colic, inferior mesenteric lymph nodes

Sigmoid colon (Fig.146)
> left colic, inferior mesenteric, sigmoid, superior rectal (haemorrhoidal), rectosigmoid lymph nodes

Rectum (Fig. 147)
> superior, middle, and inferior rectal (haemorrhoidal), inferior mesenteric, internal iliac, mesorectal (pararectal), lateral sacral, presacral, sacral promotory (Gerota) lymph nodes

Metastasis in nodes other than those listed above is classified as distant metastasis except the primary tumour directly invades other segments of colon and rectum, or the small intestine.

Fig. 139

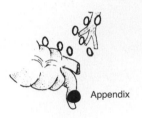

Appendix

Fig. 140

Caecum

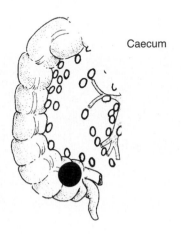

Fig. 141

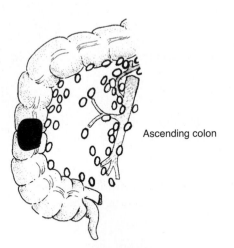

Ascending colon

Colon and Rectum

Hepatic flexure **Fig. 142**

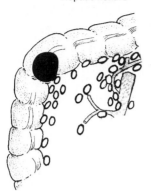

Transverse colon **Fig. 143**

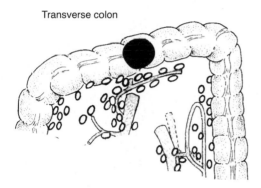

Splenic flexure   **Fig. 144**

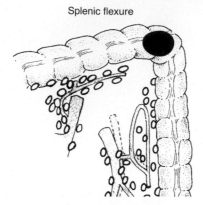

Descending colon   **Fig. 145**

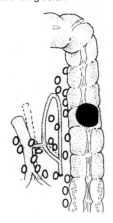

Sigmoid colon   **Fig. 146**

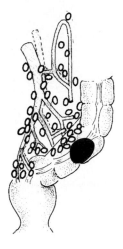

Rectum   **Fig. 147**

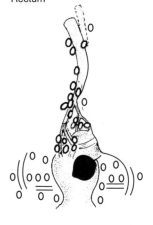

TNM Clinical Classification

T – Primary Tumour

TX   Primary tumour cannot be assessed
T0   No evidence of primary tumour
Tis   Carcinoma in situ: intraepithelial or invasion of lamina propria[1]

T1   Tumour invades submucosa (Fig. 148)
T2   Tumour invades muscularis propria (Fig. 149)

Notes
[1] Tis includes cancer cells confined within the glandular basement membrane (intraepithelial) or lamina propria (intramucosal) with no extension through muscularis mucosae into submucosa.

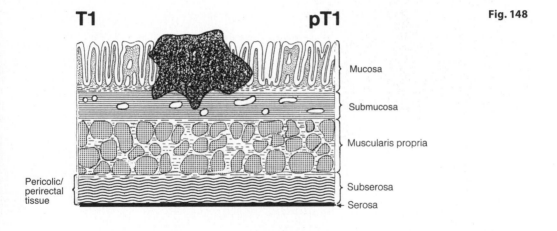

T1   **pT1**

Mucosa

Submucosa

Muscularis propria

Pericolic/perirectal tissue

Subserosa

Serosa

Fig. 148

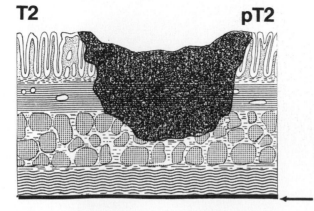

T2   **pT2**

Fig. 149

T3   Tumour invades through muscularis propria into subserosa or into non-peritoneal-
      ized pericoloic or perirectal tissues (Fig. 150)

T4   Tumour directly invades other organs or structures[2,3] and/or perforates visceral peri-
      toneum (Figs. 151, 152)

Notes

[2] Direct invasion in T4 includes invasion of other segments of the colorectum by way of the serosa, e.g., invasion of sigmoid colon by a carcinoma of the caecum.

[3] Tumour that is adherent to other organs or structures macroscopically is classified T4; however, if no tumour is present in the adhesion microscopically, the classification would be pT3.

T3   pT3

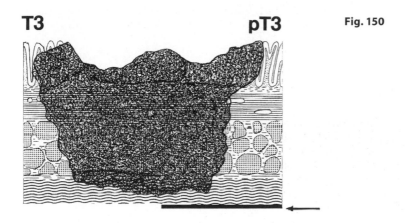

Fig. 150

T4   pT4

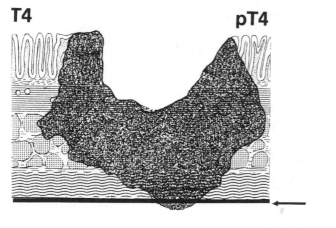

Fig. 151

T4

pT4

Fig. 152 a–c

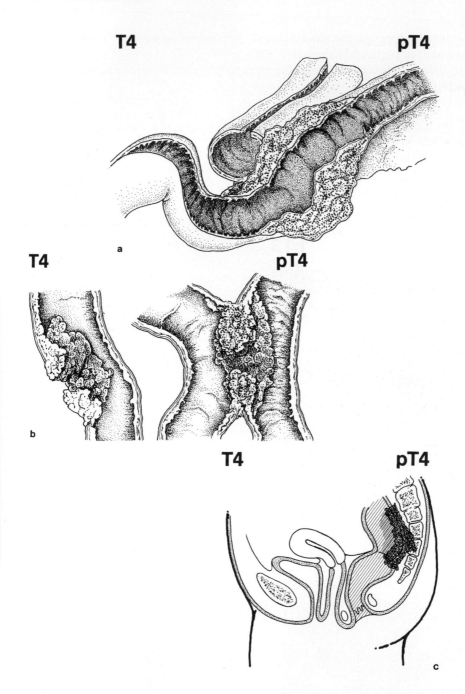

T4

pT4

a

T4

pT4

b

T4

pT4

c

N – Regional Lymph Nodes

NX   Regional lymph nodes cannot be assessed
N0   No regional lymph node metastasis

N1   Metastasis in 1 to 3 regional lymph nodes (Fig. 153)
N2   Metastasis in 4 or more regional lymph nodes (Figs. 154–156)

Note

A tumour nodule in pericolic/perirectal adipose tissue of a primary carcinoma without histological evidence of a residual lymph node in the nodule is classified in the pN category as regional lymph node metastasis if the nodule has the form and smooth contour of a lymph node. If the nodule has an irregular contour, it should be classified in the pT category and also coded as V1 (microscopic venous invasion) or V2, if it was grossly evident, because there is a strong likelihood that it represents venous invasion.

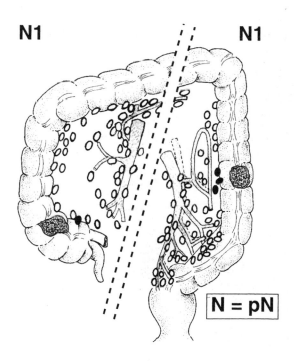

Fig. 153

N2

N2

Fig. 154

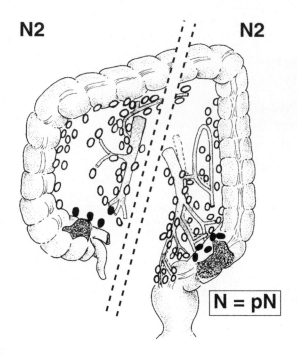

N = pN

N2

N2

Fig. 155

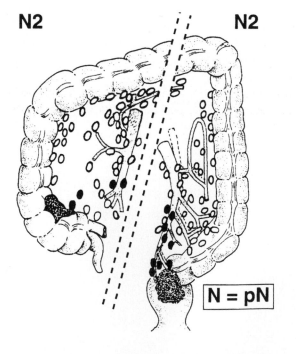

N = pN

N2

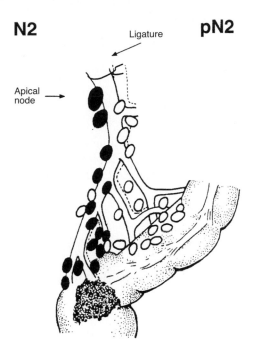

Ligature

pN2

Fig. 156
Apical node involvement does not alter
the classification

Apical
node →

pTN Pathological Classification

The pT and pN categories correspond to the T and N categories.

pN0 Histological examination of a regional lymphadenectomy specimen will ordinarily include 12 or more lymph nodes. If the examined lymph nodes are negative, but the number ordinarily resected is not met, classify as pN0.

Anal Canal (ICD-O C21.1, 2)

The anal canal (Fig. 157) extends from rectum to perianal skin (to the junction with hair-bearing skin). It is lined by the mucous membrane overlying the internal sphincter, including the transitional epithelium and dentate line. Tumours of anal margin (ICD-O C44.5) are classified with skin tumours (p. 191 ff.).

Rules for Classification

The classification applies only to carcinomas. There should be histological confirmation of the disease.

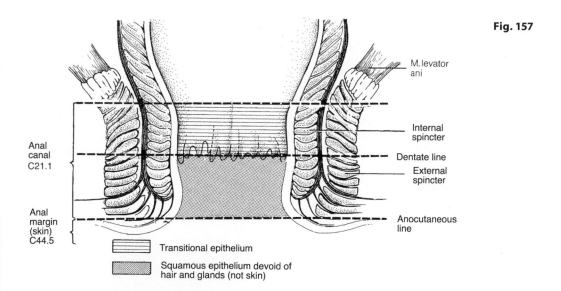

Fig. 157

M. levator ani

Internal spincter

Anal canal C21.1

Dentate line

External spincter

Anal margin (skin) C44.5

Anocutaneous line

Transitional epithelium

Squamous epithelium devoid of hair and glands (not skin)

Regional Lymph Nodes (Fig. 158)

The regional lymph nodes are the perirectal (1), the internal iliac (2), and the inguinal (3) lymph nodes.

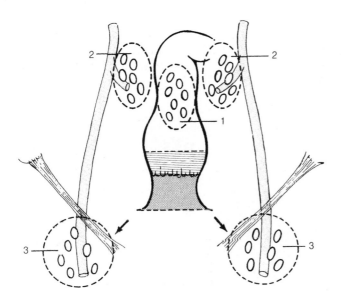

Fig. 158

TNM Clinical Classification

T – Primary Tumour

TX   Primary tumour cannot be assessed
T0   No evidence of primary tumour
Tis   Carcinoma in situ

T1   Tumour 2 cm or less in greatest dimension (Fig. 159)
T2   Tumour more than 2 cm but not more than 5 cm in greatest dimension (Fig. 160)
T3   Tumour more than 5 cm in greatest dimension (Fig. 161)

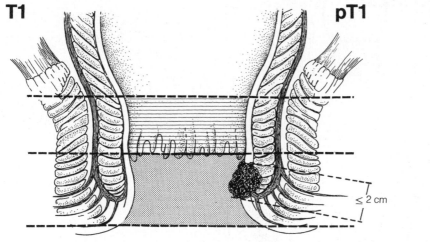

T1   **pT1**   **Fig. 159**

≤ 2 cm

T2   **T2**   **Fig. 160**

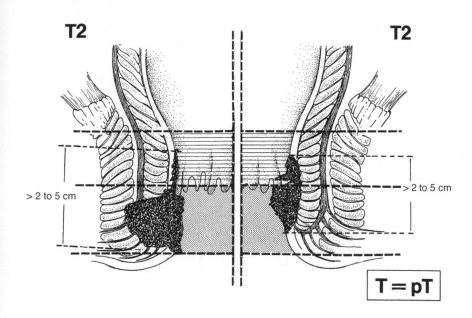

> 2 to 5 cm

> 2 to 5 cm

$$T = pT$$

T3   **pT3**   **Fig. 161**

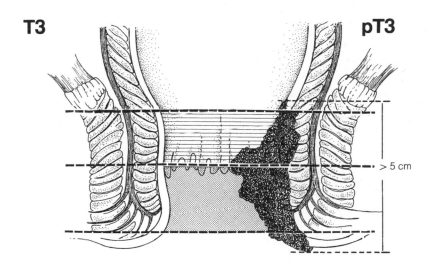

> 5 cm

T4   Tumour of any size invades adjacent organ(s), e.g., vagina, urethra, bladder (Fig. 162)

Note
Direct invasion of the rectal wall, perianal skin, subcutaneous tissue or the sphincter muscle(s) alone is not classified as T4.

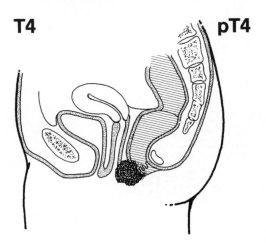

T4   **pT4**   **Fig. 162**

N – Regional Lymph Nodes

NX   Regional lymph nodes cannot be assessed
N0   No regional lymph node metastasis
N1   Metastasis in perirectal lymph node(s) (Fig. 163)

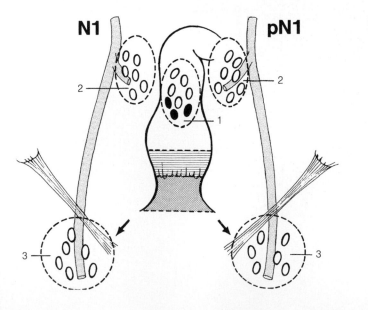

N1   **pN1**   **Fig. 163**

N2   Metastasis in unilateral internal iliac and/or inguinal lymph node(s) (Figs. 164, 165)

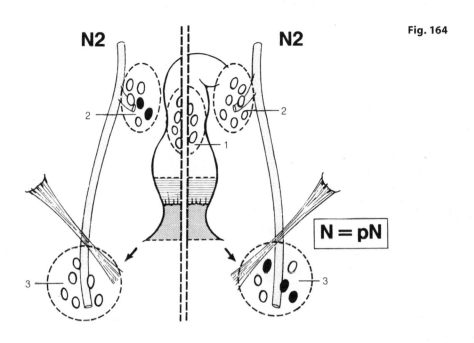

Fig. 164

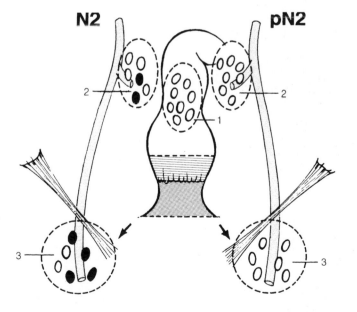

Fig. 165

N3   Metastasis in perirectal and inguinal lymph nodes and/or bilateral internal iliac and/or bilateral inguinal lymph nodes (Figs. 166–168)

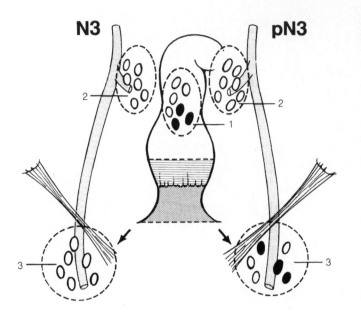

Fig. 166

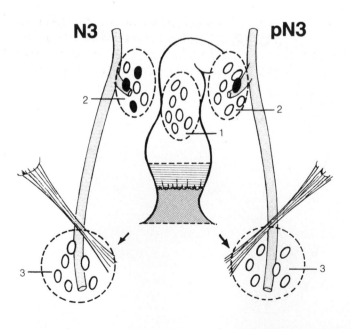

Fig. 167

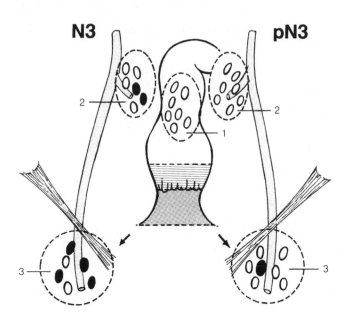

N3 **pN3**

Fig. 168

pTN Pathological Classification

The pT and pN categories correspond to the T and N categories.

pN0 Histological examination of a regional perirectal-pelvic lymphadenectomy specimen will ordinarily include 12 or more lymph nodes; histological examination of an inguinal lymphadenectomy specimen will ordinarily include 6 or more lymph nodes. If the examined lymph nodes are negative, but the number ordinarily resected is not met, classify as pN0.

Liver (ICD-O C22)

Rules for Classification

The classification is intended primarily for hepatocellular carcinoma. It may also be used for cholangio- (intrahepatic bilde duct) carcinoma of the liver. There should be histological confirmation of the disease and division of cases by histological type.

Anatomical Subsites

1. Liver (C22.0)
2. Intrahepatic bile duct (C22.1)

Regional Lymph Nodes (Fig. 169)

The regional lymph nodes are the hilar, hepatic (along the proper hepatic artery), periportal (along the portal vein) nodes and those along the abdominal inferior vena cava above the renal vein (except the inferior phrenic nodes).

Fig. 169

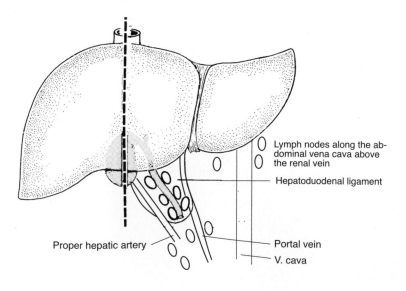

Lymph nodes along the abdominal vena cava above the renal vein

Hepatoduodenal ligament

Proper hepatic artery

Portal vein

V. cava

TN Clinical Classification

T – Primary Tumour

TX   Primary tumour cannot be assessed
T0   No evidence of primary tumour

T1   Solitary tumour without vascular invasion (Fig. 170)

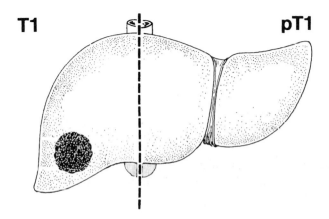

T1   **pT1**   **Fig. 170**

T2   Solitary tumour with vascular invasion; *or* multiple tumours none more than 5 cm in greatest dimension (Figs. 171, 172)

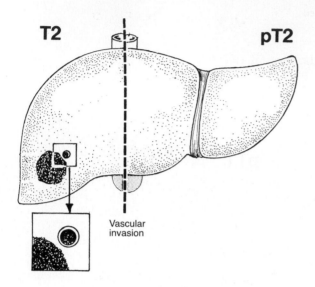

Fig. 171

Vascular
invasion

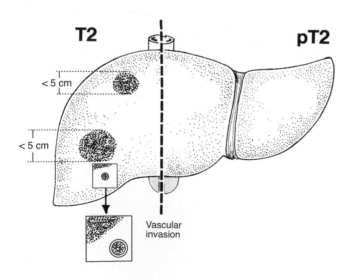

Fig. 172

< 5 cm

< 5 cm

Vascular
invasion

T3 Multiple tumours more than 5 cm or tumour involving a major branch of the portal or hepatic vein(s) (Figs. 173–175)

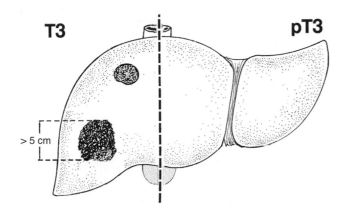

Fig. 173

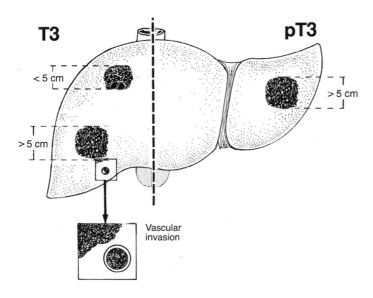

Fig. 174

Liver

T3   **pT3**   **Fig. 175**

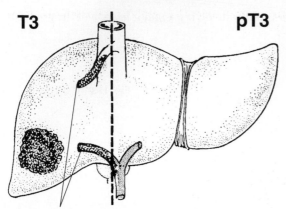

Major branch of the portal or hepatic vein (s)

T4   Tumour(s) with direct invasion of other organs other than gallbladder *or* with perforation of visceral peritoneum (Fig. 176)

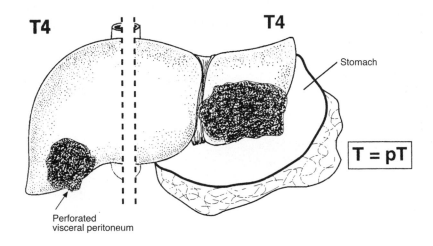

Fig. 176

N – Regional Lymph Nodes

NX   Regional lymph nodes cannot be assessed
N0   No regional lymph node metastasis
N1   Regional lymph node metastasis

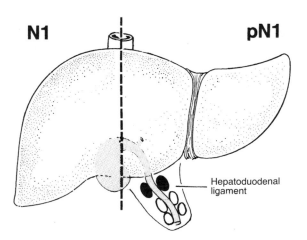

Fig. 177

pTN Pathological Classification

The pT and pN categories correspond to the T and N categories.

pN0 Histological examination of a regional lymphadenectomy specimen will ordinarily include 3 or more lymph nodes. If the examined lymph nodes are negative, but the number ordinarily resected is not met, classify as pN0.

Gallbladder (ICD-O C23)

Rules for Classification

The classification applies only to carcinomas. There should be histological confirmation of the disease.

Regional Lymph Nodes (Fig. 178)

The regional lymph nodes are the cystic duct node and the pericholedochal, hilar, peripancreatic (head only), periduodenal, periportal, coeliac, and superior mesenteric nodes.

Fig. 178

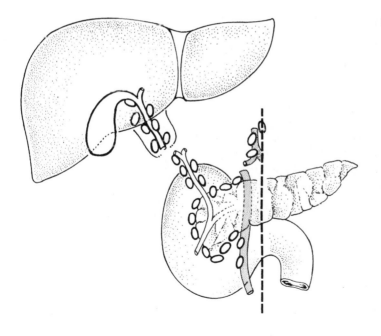

TNM Clinical Classification

T – Primary Tumour

TX   Primary tumour cannot be assessed
T0   No evidence of primary tumour
Tis   Carcinoma in situ

T1   Tumour invades lamina propria or muscle layer (Fig. 179)
T1a   Tumour invades lamina propria
T1b   Tumour invades muscle layer

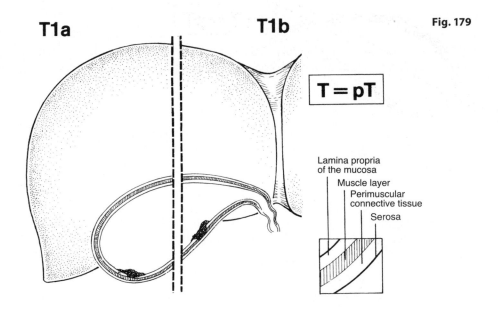

T1a   **T1b**   Fig. 179

T = pT

Lamina propria
of the mucosa
Muscle layer
Perimuscular
connective tissue
Serosa

T2   Tumour invades perimuscular connective tissue, no extension beyond serosa or into liver (Fig. 180)

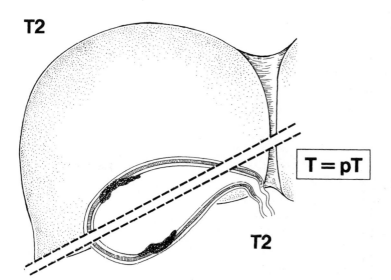

T2

Fig. 180

$T = pT$

T2

T3   Tumour perforates serosa (visceral peritoneum) and/or directly invades the liver and/or one other adjacent organ or structure, e.g., stomach, duodenum, colon, pancreas, omentum, extrahepatic bile ducts (Figs. 181, 182)

Gallbladder

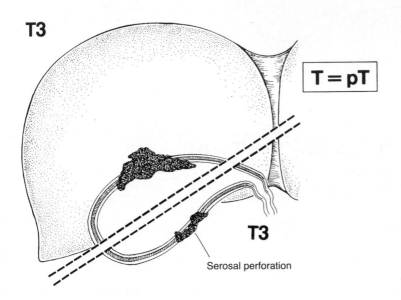

Fig. 181

T3

T = pT

T3

Serosal perforation

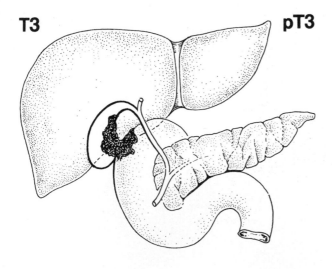

Fig. 182

T3   pT3

T4   Tumour invades main portal vein or hepatic artery, or invades two or more extrahepatic organs or structures (Figs. 183, 184)

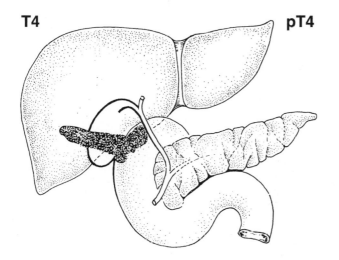

Fig. 183
Invasion of duodenum
and extrahepatic bile duct

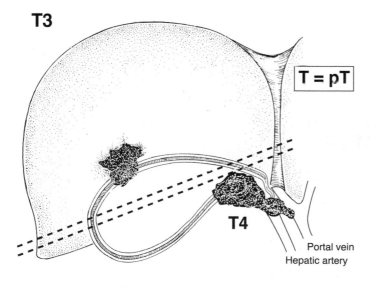

Fig. 184

Portal vein
Hepatic artery

N – Regional Lymph Nodes (Figs. 185,186)

NX   Regional lymph nodes cannot be assessed
N0   No regional lymph node metastasis
▎N1   Regional lymph node metastasis

N1   **pN1**   Fig. 185

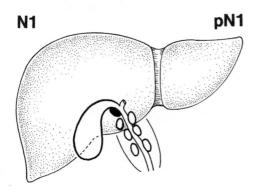

N1   Fig. 186

pN1

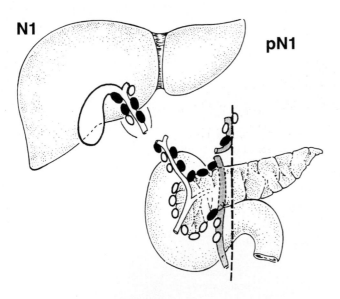

pTN Pathological Classification

The pT and pN categories correspond to the T and N categories.

pN0 Histological examination of a regional lymphadenectomy specimen will ordinarily include 3 or more lymph nodes. If the examined lymph nodes are negative, but the number ordinarily resected is not met, classify as pN0.

Extrahepatic Bile Ducts (ICD-O C24.0)

Rules for Classification

The classification applies to carcinomas of extrahepatic bile ducts and those of choledochal cysts. There should be histological confirmation of the disease.

Anatomic subsites (Fig. 187)

1. Right hepatic duct
2. Left hepatic duct
3. Common hepatic duct
4. Common bile duct
5. Cystic duct

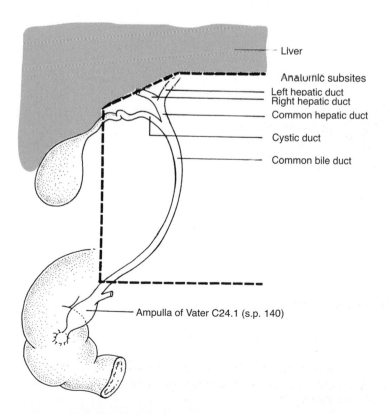

Fig. 187

Liver

Anatomic subsites
Left hepatic duct
Right hepatic duct
Common hepatic duct

Cystic duct

Common bile duct

Ampulla of Vater C24.1 (s.p. 140)

Regional Lymph Nodes (Fig.178, p. 129)

The regional lymph nodes are the cystic duct, pericholedochal, hilar, peripancreatic (head only), periduodenal, periportal, coeliac, and superior mesenteric nodes.

TN Clinical Classification

T – Primary Tumour

TX   Primary tumour cannot be assessed
T0   No evidence of primary tumour
Tis   Carcinoma in situ

T1   Tumour confined to the wall of the bile duct[1] (Fig. 188)
T2   Tumour invades beyond the wall of the bile duct (Fig. 189)

Note
[1] The "wall of the bile duct" includes epithelium, subepithelial connective tissue and the fibromuscular layer.

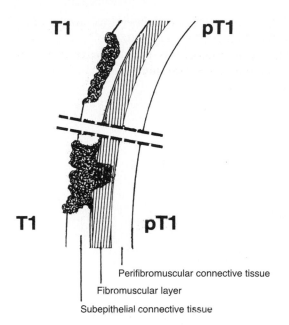

Fig. 188

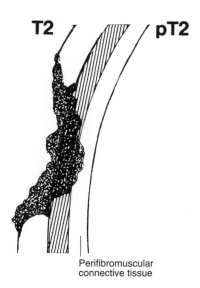

Perifibromuscular connective tissue

Fibromuscular layer

Subepithelial connective tissue

Fig. 189

Perifibromuscular
connective tissue

T3   Tumour invades the liver, gallbladder, pancreas, and/or unilateral tributaries of the portal vein (right or left) or hepatic artery (right or left) (Fig. 190)

T4   Tumour invades any of the following: main portal vein or its tributaries bilaterally, common hepatic artery, or other adjacent structures, e.g., colon, stomach, duodenum, abdominal wall (Fig. 191)

T3   **pT3**   **Fig. 190**

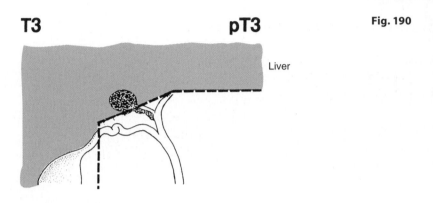

Liver

T3   **Fig. 191**

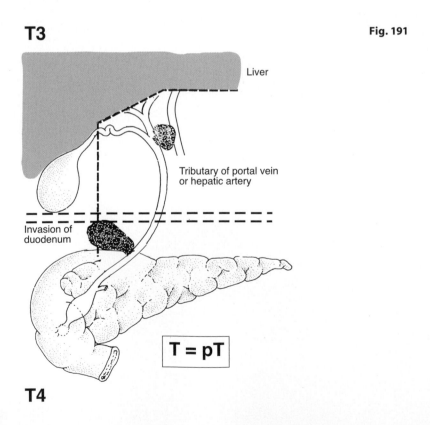

Liver

Tributary of portal vein
or hepatic artery

Invasion of
duodenum

T = pT

T4

N – Regional Lymph Nodes

NX Regional lymph nodes cannot be assessed
N0 No regional lymph node metastasis
N1 Regional lymph node metastasis (Figs. 185, 186, p. 134)

pTN Pathological Classification

The pT and pN categories correspond to the T and N categories.

pN0 Histological examination of a regional lymphadenectomy specimen will ordinarily include 3 or more lymph nodes. If the examined lymph nodes are negative, but the number ordinarily resected is not met, classify as pN0.

Ampulla of Vater (ICD-O C24.1) (Fig. 192)

Rules for Classification

The classification applies only to carcinomas. There should be histological confirmation of the disease.

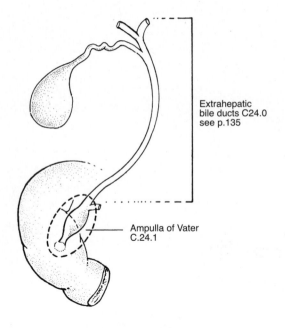

Fig. 192

Extrahepatic
bile ducts C24.0
see p.135

Ampulla of Vater
C.24.1

Regional Lymph Nodes (Fig.193)

The regional lymph nodes are:
Superior   Superior to head (1) and body (2) of pancreas
Inferior   Inferior to head (3) and body (4) of pancreas

Anterior   Anterior pancreaticoduodenal (5), pyloric (6, not shown in Fig.193) and proximal mesenteric (7)

Posterior   Posterior pancreaticoduodenal (8), common bile duct (9), and proximal mesenteric (7)

Note

The splenic lymph nodes and those of the tail of the pancreas are not regional; metastases to these lymph nodes are coded M1.

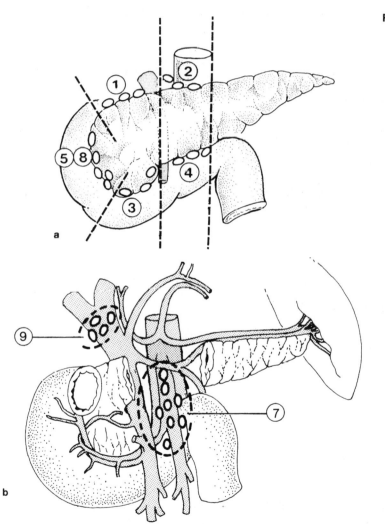

Fig. 193a, b

TNM Clinical Classification

T – Primary Tumour

TX   Primary tumour cannot be assessed
T0   No evidence of primary tumour
Tis   Carcinoma in situ

T1   Tumour limited to ampulla of Vater or sphincter of Oddi (Fig. 194)
T2   Tumour invades duodenal wall (Fig. 195)

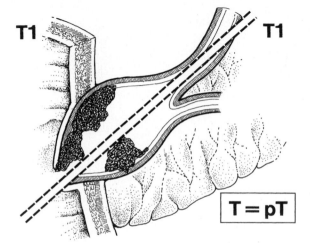

Fig. 194

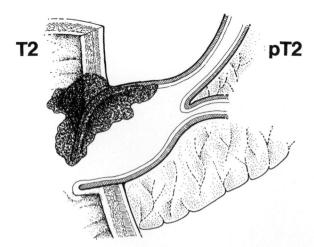

Fig. 195

T3   Tumour invades pancreas (Fig. 196)

T4   Tumour invades peripancreatic soft tissues, or other adjacent organs or structures (Fig. 197)

T3   **pT3**   **Fig. 196**

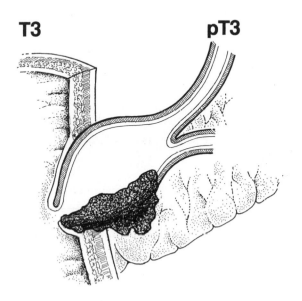

T4   **pT4**   **Fig. 197**

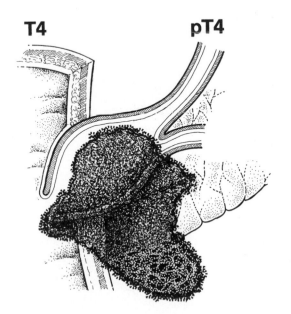

N – Regional Lymph Nodes

NX   Regional lymph nodes cannot be assessed
N0   No regional lymph node metastasis
N1   Regional lymph node metastasis (Figs. 198, 199)

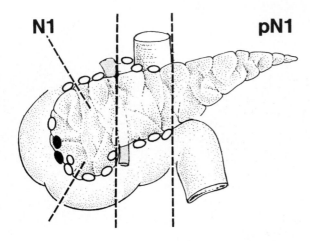

Fig. 198

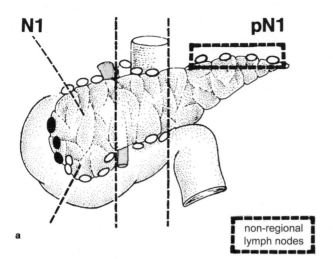

Fig. 199a, b

non-regional
lymph nodes

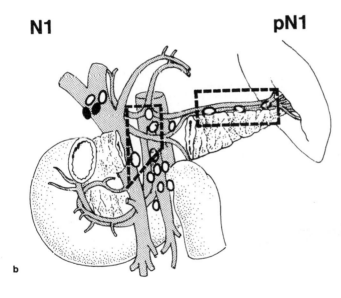

M – Distant Metastasis

MX   Distant metastasis cannot be assessed

M0   No distant metastasis

M1   Distant metastasis (Fig. 200a,b) (includes metastasis in splenic lymph nodes and/or those at the tail of the pancreas)

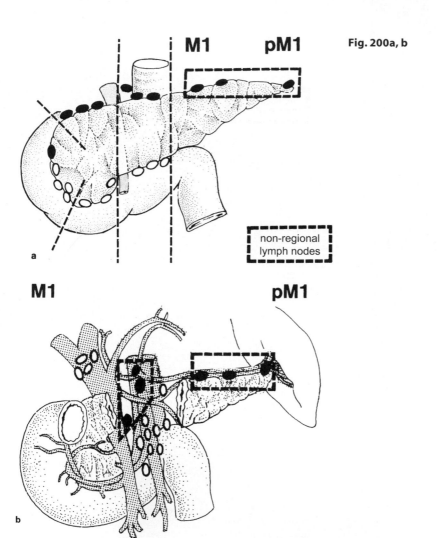

Fig. 200a, b

pTNM Pathological Classification

The pT, pN and pM categories correspond to the T, N and M categories.

pN0 Histological examination of a regional lymphadenectomy specimen will ordinarily include 10 or more lymph nodes. If the examined lymph nodes are negative, but the number ordinarily resected is not met, classify as pN0.

Pancreas (ICD-O C25)

Rules for Classification

The classification applies only to carcinomas of the exocrine pancreas. There should be histological or cytological confirmation of the disease.

Anatomical Subsites (Fig. 201)

1. Head of pancreas[1] (C25.0)
2. Body of pancreas[2] (C25.1)
3. Tail of pancreas[3] (C25.2)

Notes

[1] Tumours of the head of the pancreas are those arising to the right of the left border of the superior mesenteric vein. The uncinate process is considered as part of the head.

[2] Tumours of the body are those arising between the left border of the superior mesenteric vein and left border of the aorta.

[3] Tumours of the tail are those arising between the left border of the aorta and the hilum of the spleen.

Pancreas

Fig. 201

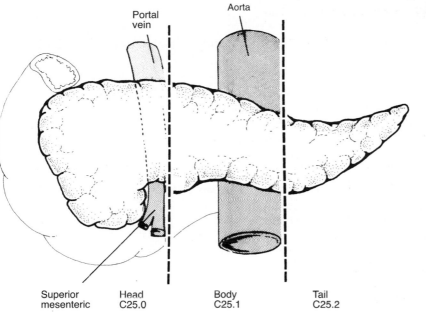

Portal
vein

Aorta

Superior
mesenteric

Head
C25.0

Body
C25.1

Tail
C25.2

Regional Lymph Nodes (Fig. 202a,b)

The regional lymph nodes are the peripancreatic nodes, which may be subdivided as follows:

Superior:	Superior to head (1) and body (2)
Inferior:	Inferior to head (3) and body (4)
Anterior:	Anterior pancreaticoduodenal (5), pyloric (for tumours of head only) (6, not shown in Fig. 202), and proximal mesenteric (7)
Posterior:	Posterior pancreaticoduodenal (8), common bile duct (9), and proximal mesenteric (7)
Splenic:	Hilum of spleen (10) and tail of pancreas (11) (for tumours of body and tail only)
Coeliac:	for tumours of head only (12)

Pancreas

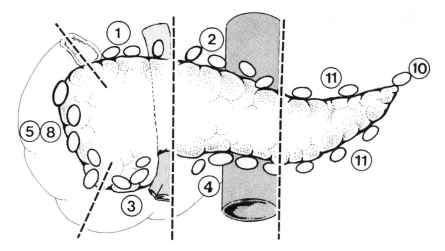

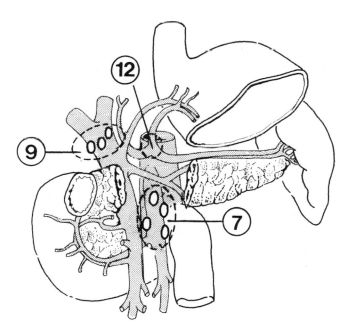

TNM Clinical Classification

T – Primary Tumour

TX   Primary tumour cannot be assessed
T0   No evidence of primary tumour
Tis Carcinoma in situ

T1   Tumour limited to the pancreas, 2 cm or less in greatest dimension (Fig. 203)
T2   Tumour limited to the pancreas, more than 2 cm in greatest dimension (Fig. 203)

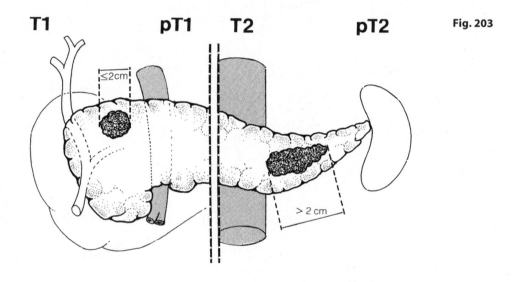

Fig. 203

T3   Tumour extends beyond pancreas, but without involvement of coeliac axis or superior mesenteric artery (Fig. 204)

T4   Tumour involves coeliac axis or superior mesenteric artery (Fig. 205)

T3   **pT3**   **Fig. 204**

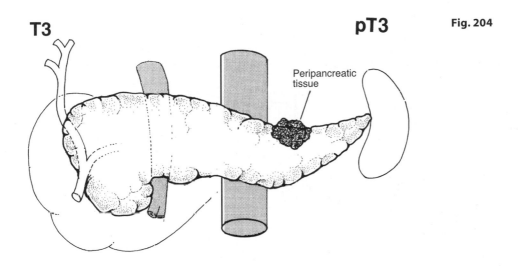

Peripancreatic tissue

T4   **pT4**   **Fig. 205**

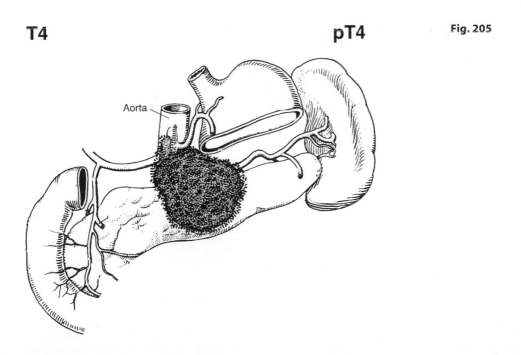

Aorta

N – Regional Lymph Nodes

NX   Regional lymph nodes cannot be assessed
N0   No regional lymph node metastasis
N1   Regional lymph node metastasis (Figs. 206, 207)

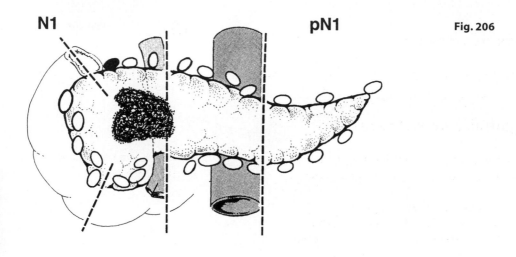

N1   **pN1**   **Fig. 206**

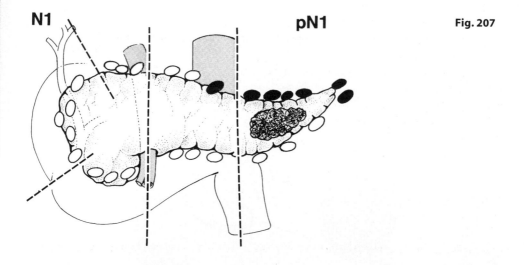

N1   **pN1**   **Fig. 207**

pTN Pathological Classification

The pT and pN categories correspond to the T and N categories.

pN0 Histological examination of a regional lymphadenectomy specimen will ordinarily include 10 or more lymph nodes. If the examined lymph nodes are negative, but the number ordinarily resected is not met, classify as pN0.

Lung and Pleural Tumours

Introductory Notes

The classifications apply to carcinomas of the lung and malignant mesothelioma of pleura.

Regional Lymph Nodes (Figs. 208, 209)

The regional lymph nodes for lung tumours are the intrathoracic, scalene, and supraclavicular nodes, for pleural mesothelioma in addition the internal mammary nodes.

The intrathoracic nodes include:
a) *Mediastinal nodes* (Figs. 208, 209)
- (1) highest (superior) mediastinal
- (2) paratracheal (upper tracheal)
- (3) pretracheal
- (3a) anterior mediastinal
- (3p) retrotracheal (posterior mediastinal)
- (4) tracheobronchial (lower paratracheal) (including azygos nodes)
- (5) subaortic (aortic window)
- (6) para-aortic (ascending aorta or phrenic)
- (7) subcarinal
- (8) paraoesophageal (below carina)
- (9) pulmonary ligament

b) *Peribronchial and hilar nodes* (Figs. 208, 209)
- (10) hilar (main bronchus)
- (11) interlobar
- (12) lobar
- (13) segmental
- (14) subsegmental

Direct extension of the primary tumour into lymph nodes is classified as lymph node metastasis.

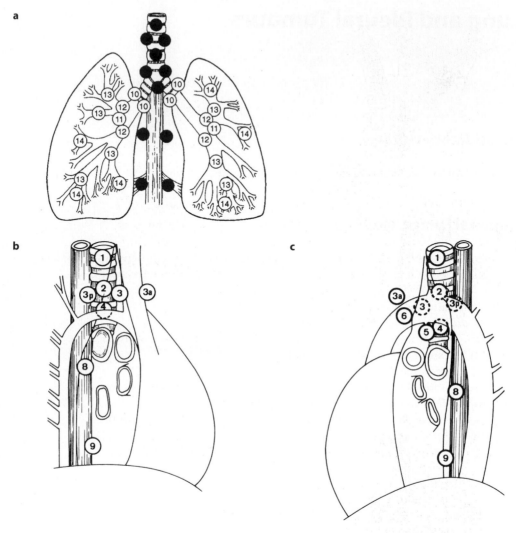

Fig. 208a–c. Lymph node map of Naruke. [Modified from Naruke T, Suemasu K, Ishikawa S (1978) Lymph node mapping and curability at various levels of metastasis in resected lung cancer. J Thorac Cardiovasc Surg 76: 832–839]

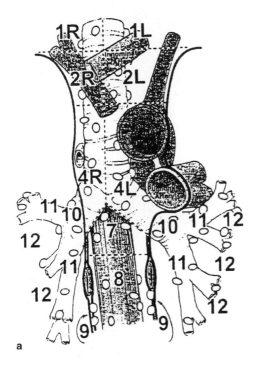

a

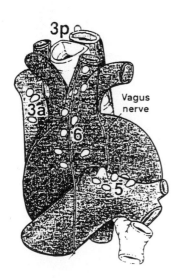

b

N2 Lymph Nodes

**Superior mediastinal
lymph nodes**

1. Highest mediastinal

2. Upper paratracheal

3. Pre- and retrotracheal

4. Lower paratracheal
   (including Azygos
   nodes)

Aortic lymph nodes

5. Subaortic (A-P windows)

6. Paraaortic (ascending
   aorta or phrenic)

**Inferior mediastinal
lymph nodes**

7. Subcarinal

8. Paraoesophageal
   (below carina)

9. Pulmonary ligament

N1 Lymph nodes

10. Hilar

11. Interlobar

12. Lobar

13. Segmental

14. Subsegmental

Fig. 209a, b. Regional lymph nodes for lung cancer. Used with the permission of the American Joint Committee on Cancer (AJCC), Chicago, Illinois. The original source for the material is the AJCC Cancer Staging Manual, 6th edition (2002) Greene FL, Page DL, Fleming ID, Fritz AG, Balch CM, Haller DG Morrow M (eds) Springer, New York.

Lung (ICD-O C34)

Rules for Classification

The classification applies only to carcinomas. There should be histological confirmation of the disease and division of cases by histological type.

Anatomical Subsites (Fig. 210)

1. Main bronchus (C34.0)
2. Upper lobe (C34.1)
3. Middle lobe (C34.2)
4. Lower lobe (C34.3)

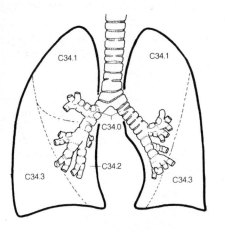

Fig. 210

Regional Lymph Nodes

The regional lymph nodes are the intrathoracic, scalene, and supraclavicular nodes (see pp. 155–157).

TNM Clinical Classification

T – Primary Tumour

TX   Primary tumour cannot be assessed, *or* tumour proven by the presence of malignant cells in sputum or bronchial washings but not visualized by imaging or bronchoscopy

T0   No evidence of primary tumour

Tis   Carcinoma in situ

T1   Tumour 3 cm or less in greatest dimension, surrounded by lung or visceral pleura, without bronchoscopic evidence of invasion more proximal than the lobar bronchus (i.e., not in the main bronchus)[1] (Fig. 211)

T2   Tumour with *any* of the following features of size or extent (Fig. 212):
   - More than 3 cm in greatest dimension
   - Involves main bronchus, 2 cm or more distal to the carina
   - Invades visceral pleura
   - Associated with atelectasis or obstructive pneu monitis – that extends to the hilar region but does not involve the entire lung

T3   Tumour of any size that directly invades any of the following: chest wall (including superior sulcus tumours), diaphragm, mediastinal pleura, parietal pericardium; *or* tumour in the main bronchus less than 2 cm distal to the carina[1] but without involvement of the carina; *or* associated atelectasis or obstructive pneumonitis of the entire lung (Fig. 213)

T4   Tumour of any size that invades any of the following: mediastinum, heart, great vessels, trachea, oesophagus, vertebral body, carina; separate tumour nodule(s) in the same lobe; tumour with malignant pleural effusion[2] (Figs. 214–222)

Notes

[1] The uncommon superficial spreading tumour of any size with its invasive component limited to the bronchial wall, which may extend proximal to the main bronchus, is also classified as T1.

[2] Most pleural effusions with lung cancer are due to tumour. In a few patients, however, multiple cytopathological examinations of pleural fluid are negative for tumour, and the fluid is non-bloody and is not an exudate. Where these elements and clinical judgment dictate that the effusion is not related to the tumour, the effusion should be excluded as a staging element and the patient should be classified as T1, T2, or T3.

Lung

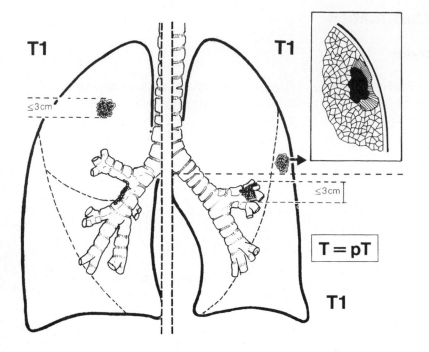

Fig. 211

T1

T1

≤3 cm

≤3 cm

T = pT

T1

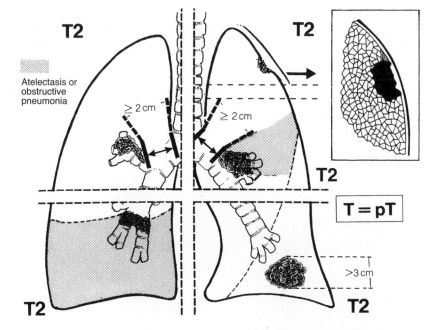

Fig. 212

T2

T2

Atelectasis or
obstructive
pneumonia

≥ 2 cm

≥ 2 cm

T2

T = pT

>3 cm

T2

T2

Fig. 213

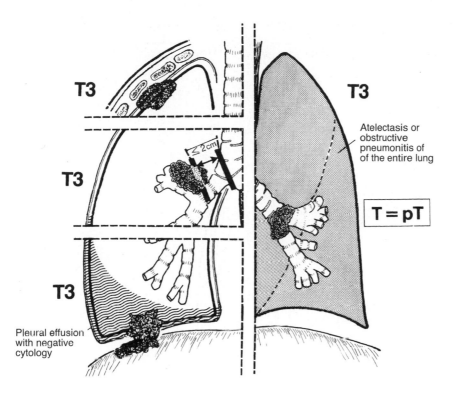

T3

T3

T3

Pleural effusion
with negative
cytology

T3

Atelectasis or
obstructive
pneumonitis of
of the entire lung

T = pT

Fig. 214

T4

pT4

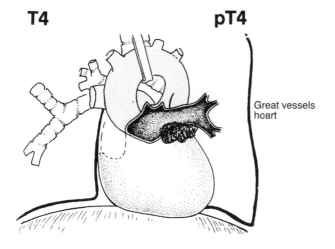

Great vessels
heart

Lung

T4   **pT4**   **Fig. 215**

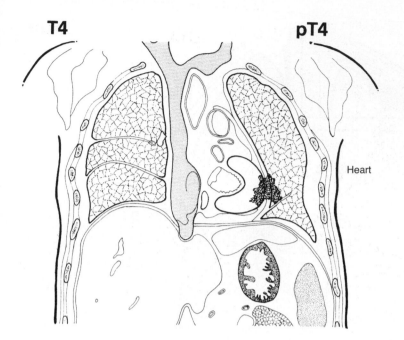

Heart

T4   **pT4**   **Fig. 216**

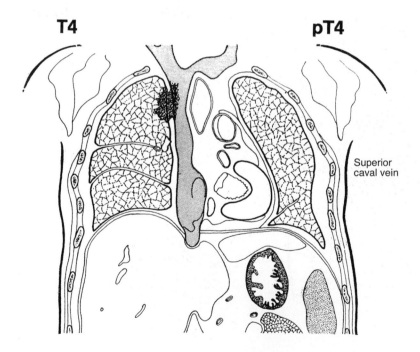

Superior
caval vein

Fig. 217

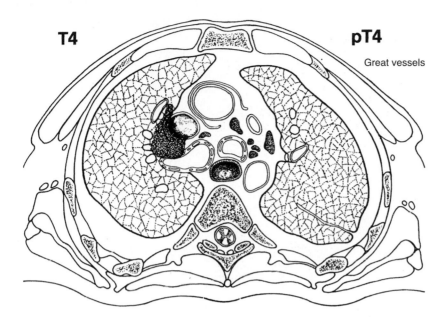

T4   pT4

Great vessels

Fig. 218

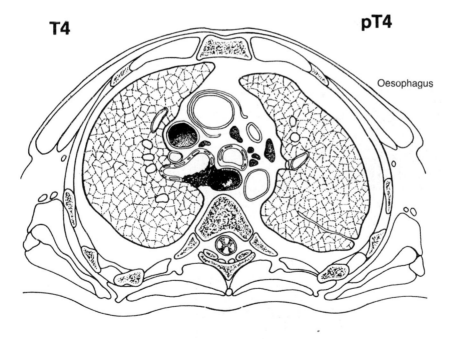

T4   pT4

Oesophagus

Lung

T4   pT4   Fig. 219

Vertebral
body

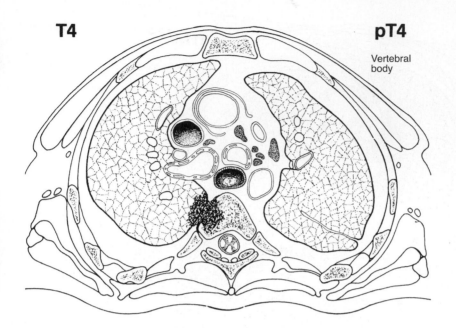

T4   M1   Fig. 220

T = pT

M = pM

Primary
tumour

Primary
tumour

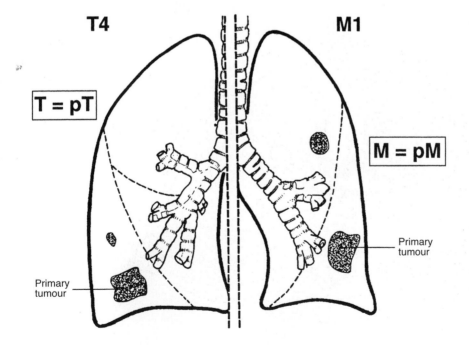

T4

pT4

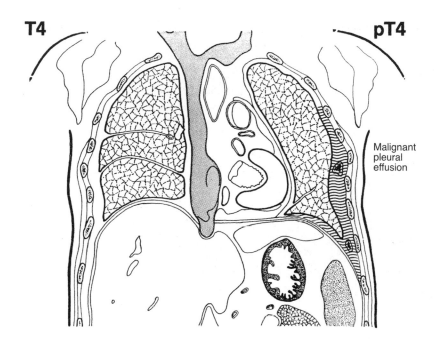

Malignant
pleural
effusion

Fig. 221

T4

pT4

Malignant
pleura
effusion

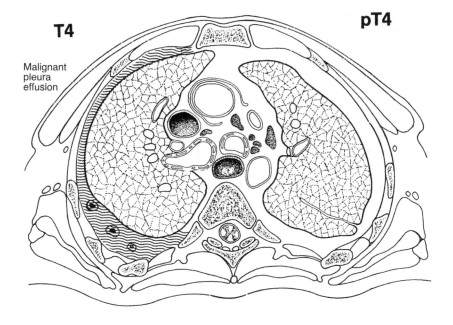

Fig. 222

N – Regional Lymph Nodes

NX   Regional lymph nodes cannot be assessed
N0   No regional lymph node metastasis
N1   Metastasis in ipsilateral peribronchial and/or ipsilateral hilar lymph nodes and intrapulmonary nodes, including involvement by direct extension (Fig. 223)

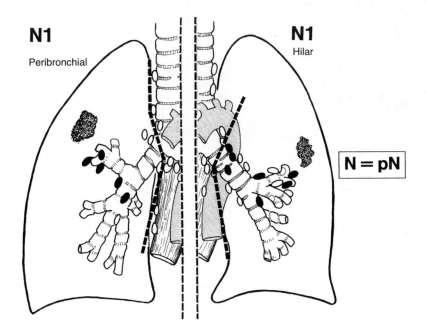

Fig. 223

N1
Peribronchial

N1
Hilar

N = pN

N2   Metastasis in ipsilateral mediastinal and/or subcarinal lymph node(s) (Fig. 224)

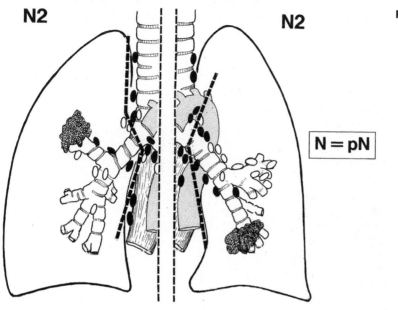

Fig. 224

Lung

N3   Metastasis in contralateral mediastinal, contralateral hilar, ipsilateral or contralateral scalene, or supraclavicular lymph node(s) (Fig. 225)

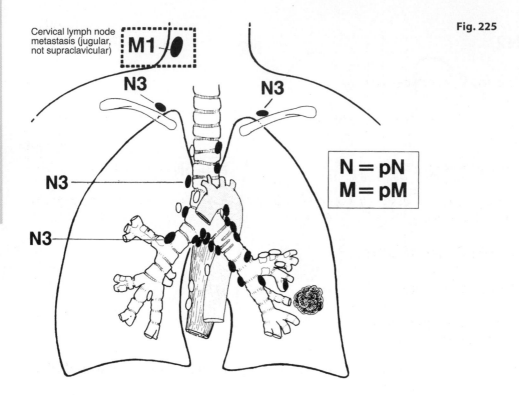

Fig. 225

Cervical lymph node metastasis (jugular, not supraclavicular)

M1

N3   N3

N3

N3

N = pN
M = pM

M – Distant Metastasis

MX   Distant metastasis cannot be assessed
M0   No distant metastasis
M1   Distant metastasis, includes separate tumour nodule(s) in a different lobe (ipsilateral or contralateral) (Figs. 220, 225)

pTNM Pathological Classification

The pT, pN, and pM categories correspond to the T, N, and M categories.

pN0 Histological examination of hilar and mediastinal lymphadenectomy specimen(s) will ordinarily include 6 or more lymph nodes. If the examined lymph nodes are negative, but the number ordinarily resected is not met, classify as pN0. The number of lymph nodes should be recorded in the pathology report.

Pleural Mesothelioma (ICD-O C38.4)

Rules for Classification

The classification applies only to malignant mesothelioma of the pleura. There should be histological confirmation of the disease.

Regional Lymph Nodes

The regional lymph nodes are the intrathoracic, internal mammary, scalene, and supraclavicular nodes (see pp. 155–157).

TN Clinical Classification

T – Primary Tumour

TX   Primary tumour cannot be assessed
T0   No evidence of primary tumour

T1   Tumour involves ipsilateral parietal pleura with or without focal involvement of visceral pleura (Fig. 226)
       T1a   Tumour involves ipsilateral parietal (mediastinal, diaphragmatic) pleura. No involvement of visceral pleura (Fig. 226)
       T1b   Tumour involves ipsilateral parietal (mediastinal, diaphragmatic) pleura, with focal involvement of visceral pleura (Fig. 226)

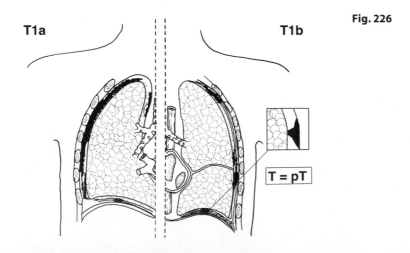

Fig. 226

T1a   T1b

T = pT

T2   Tumour involves any of the ipsilateral pleural surfaces, with at least one of the following:
- confluent visceral pleural tumour including the fissurae (Fig. 227)
- invasion of diaphragmatic muscle (Fig. 228)
- invasion of lung parenchyma (Fig. 229)

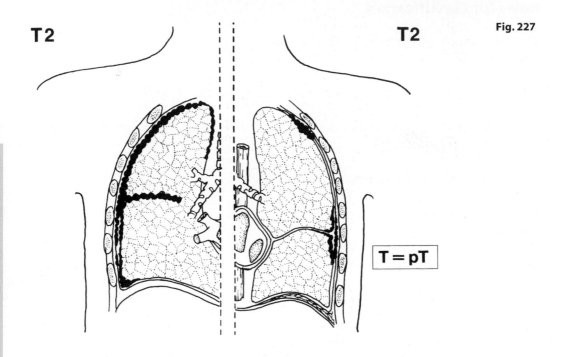

T2

T2

Fig. 227

T = pT

T2

T2

Fig. 228

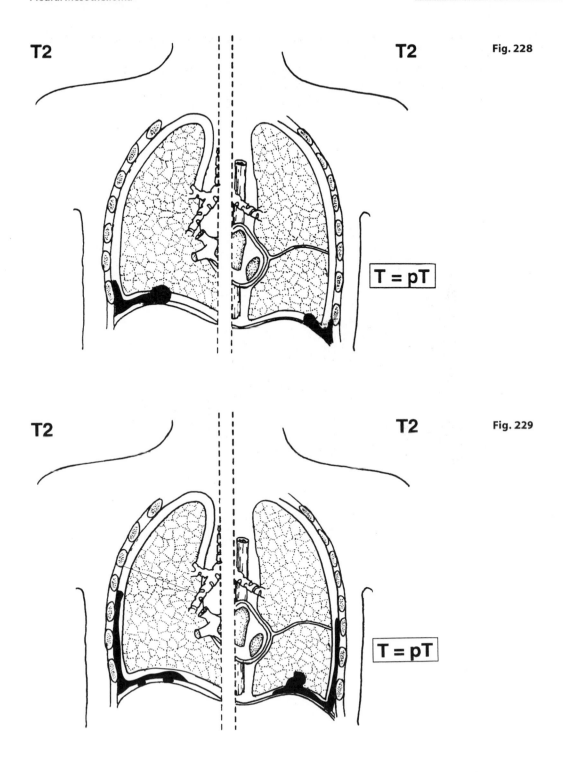

$\boxed{\text{T = pT}}$

T2

T2

Fig. 229

$\boxed{\text{T = pT}}$

T3*   Tumour involves any of the ipsilateral pleural surfaces, with at least one of the following:
- invasion of endothoracic fascia (Fig. 230)
- invasion of mediastinal fat (Fig. 231)
- solitary focus of tumour invading soft tissue of the chest wall (Fig. 230)
- non-transmural involvement of pericardium (Fig. 231)

Note
see p. 174

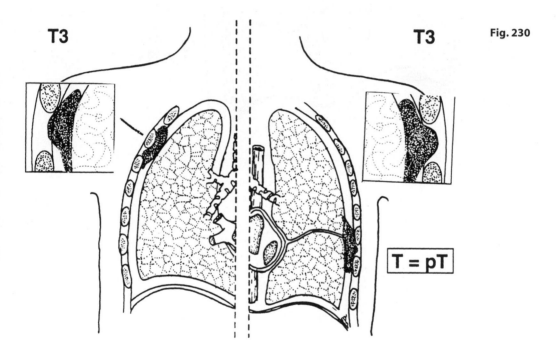

Fig. 230

Fig. 231

T3

T3

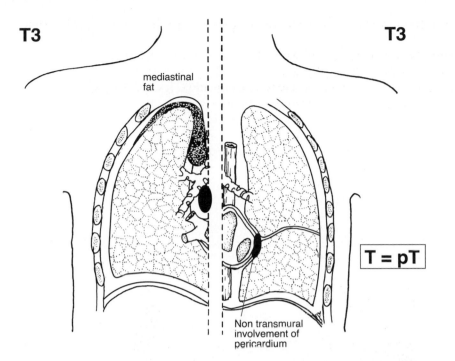

mediastinal
fat

Non transmural
involvement of
pericardium

$T = pT$

T4**   Tumour involves any of the ipsilateral pleural surfaces, with at least one of the following:
- diffuse or multifocal invasion of soft tissues of the chest wall (Fig. 232)
- any involvement of rib (Fig. 232)
- invasion through the diaphragm to the peritoneum (Figs. 233, 235)
- invasion of any mediastinal organ(s) (Fig. 234)
- direct extension to contralateral pleura (Fig. 235)
- invasion into the spine (Fig. 234)
- extension to the internal surface of the pericardium (Fig. 234)
- pericardial effusion with positive cytology
- invasion of the myocardium (Fig. 235)
- invasion of the brachial plexus (Fig. 233)

Notes
*   T3 describes locally advanced, but potentially resectable tumour
**   T4 describes locally advanced, technically unresectable tumour

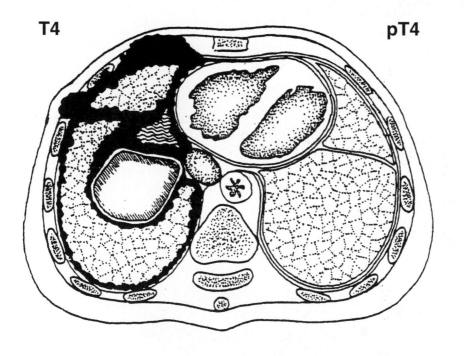

T4   pT4   Fig. 232

T4 **pT4** **Fig. 233**

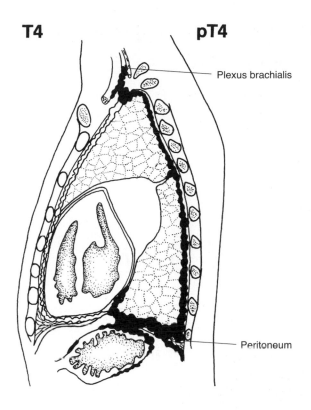

Plexus brachialis

Peritoneum

T4 **pT4** **Fig. 234**

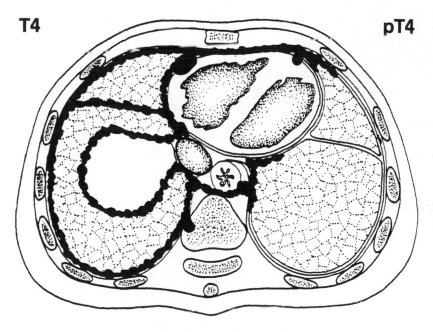

Direct extension to contralateral pleura

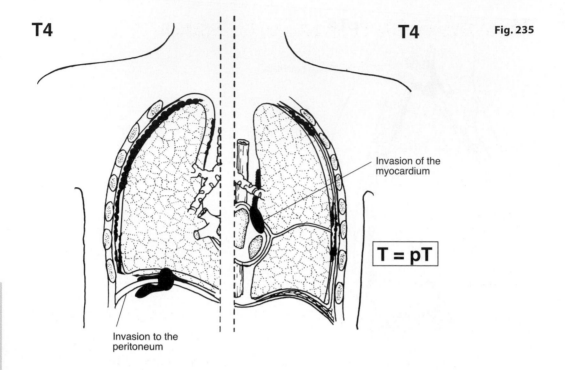

T4   **T4**   Fig. 235

Invasion of the myocardium

T = pT

Invasion to the peritoneum

N – Regional Lymph Nodes

NX   Regional lymph nodes cannot be assessed
N0   No regional lymph node metastasis

N1   Metastasis in ipsilateral peribronchial and/or ipsilateral hilar lymph nodes, including involvement by direct extension (Fig. 223, p. 166)
N2   Metastasis in subcarinal lymph node(s) and /or ipsilateral internal mammary or mediastinal lymph node(s)
N3   Metastasis in contralateral mediastinal, internal mammary, or hilar node(s) and /or ipsilateral or contralateral supraclavicular or scalene lymph node(s)

pTN Pathological Classification

The pT and pN categories correspond to the T and N categories.

Tumours of Bone and Soft Tissues

Introductory Notes

The following sites are included:

- Bone
- Soft tissue

Regional Lymph Nodes

The regional lymph nodes are those appropriate to the site of the primary tumour. Regional lymph node metastasis are rare.

The definitions of the N categories for all tumours of bone and soft tissues are:

N – Regional Lymph Nodes

NX   Regional lymph nodes cannot be assessed
N0   No regional lymph node metastasis
N1   Regional lymph node metastasis

one

Bone (ICD-O C40, 41)

Rules for Classification

The classification applies to all primary malignant bone tumours except malignant lymphomas, multiple myeloma, surface/juxtacortical osteosarcoma, and juxtacortical chondrosarcoma. There should be histological confirmation of the disease and division of cases by histological type and grade.

TNM Clinical Classification

T – Primary Tumour

TX   Primary tumour cannot be assessed
T0   No evidence of primary tumour

T1   Tumour 8 cm or less in greatest dimension (Fig. 236)
T2   Tumour more than 8 cm in greatest dimension (Fig. 237)
T3   Discontinuous tumours in the primary bone site (Fig. 238)

T1   **pT1**   **Fig. 236**

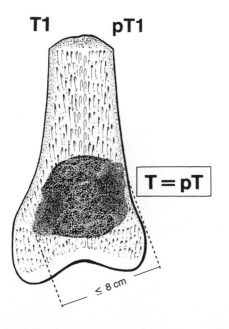

T = pT

≤ 8 cm

T2　　　pT2

Fig. 237

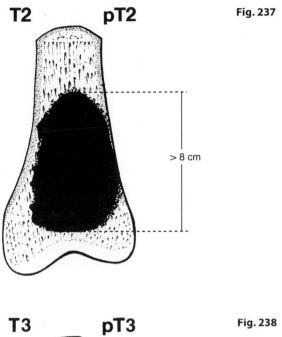

> 8 cm

T3　　　pT3

Fig. 238

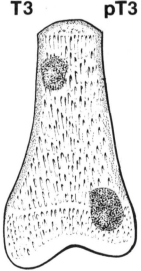

pTN Pathological Classification

The pT and pN categories correspond to the T and N categories.

Soft Tissues (ICD-O C38.1–3, C47–49)

Rules for Classification

There should be histological confirmation of the disease and division of cases by histological type and grade.

Anatomical Sites and Subsites

1. Connective, subcutaneous, and other soft tissues (C49), peripheral nerves (C47)
2. Retroperitoneum (C48)
3. Mediastinum: anterior (38.1), posterior (C38.2), mediastinum, NOS (C38.3)

Histological Types of Tumour

The following histological types of malignant tumour are included, the appropriate ICD-O morphology rubrics being indicated:

Alveolar soft part sarcoma	9581/3
Epithelioid sarcoma	8804/3
Extraskeletal chondrosarcoma	9220/3
Extraskeletal osteosarcoma	9180/3
Extraskeletal EWING's sarcoma	9260/3
Primitive neuroectodermal tumour (PNET)	9473/3
Fibrosarcoma	8810/3
Leiomyosarcoma	8890/3
Liposarcoma	8850/3
Malignant fibrous histiocytoma	8830/3
Malignant hemangiopericytoma	9150/3
Malignant mesenchymoma	8990/3
Malignant peripheral nerve sheath tumour	9540/3
Rhabdomyosarcoma	8900/3
Synovial sarcoma	9040/3
Sarcoma NOS (not otherwise specified)	8800/3

The following histological types are not included: Kaposi sarcoma, dermatofibrosarcoma (protuberans), fibromatosis (desmoid tumour), and sarcoma arising from the dura mater, brain, hollow viscera, or parenchymatous organs (with the exception of breast sarcomas). Angiosarcoma, an aggressive sarcoma, is excluded because its natural history is not consistent with the classification.

T Clinical Classification

T – Primary Tumour

TX   Primary tumour cannot be assessed
T0   No evidence of primary tumour

T1   Tumour 5 cm or less in greatest dimension
      T1a   Superficial tumour* (Fig. 239)
      T1b   Deep tumour* (Fig. 240)
T2   Tumour more than 5 cm in greatest dimension
      T2a   Superficial tumour* (Fig. 239)
      T2b   Deep tumour* (Fig. 240)

Note
* Superficial tumour is located exclusively above the superficial fascia without invasion of the fascia; deep tumour is located either exclusively beneath the superficial fascia or superficial to the fascia with invasion of or through the fascia. Retroperitoneal, mediastinal, and pelvic sarcomas are classified as deep tumours.

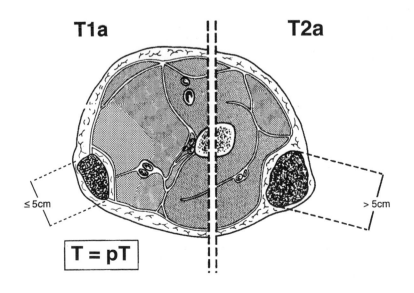

T1a   **T2a**   Fig. 239

≤5cm   > 5cm

T = pT

T1b   pT1b

Fig. 240

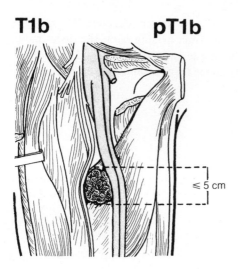

≤ 5 cm

T2b   pT2b

Fig. 241

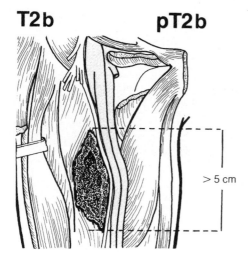

> 5 cm

pT Pathological Classification

The pT categories correspond to the T categories.

Skin Tumours

Introductory Notes

The classifications apply to carcinomas of the skin, excluding eyelid (see p. 341), vulva (see p. 225), and penis (see p. 275) and to malignant melanomas of the skin including eyelid.

Anatomical Sites

The following sites are identified by ICD-O topography rubrics:

- Lip (excluding vermilion surface) (C44.0)
- Eyelid (C44.1)
- External ear (C44.2)
- Other and unspecified parts of face (C44.3)
- Scalp and neck (C44.4)
- Trunk including anal margin and perianal skin (C44.5)
- Upper limb and shoulder (C44.6)
- Lower limb and hip (C44.7)
- Vulva (C51.0)
- Penis (C60.9)
- Scrotum (C63.2)

Regional Lymph Nodes (Figs. 242, 243a,b)

The regional lymph nodes are those appropriate to the site of the primary tumour.

Unilateral Tumours

Head, neck:	Ipsilateral preauricular, submandibular, cervical, and supraclavicular lymph nodes
Thorax:	Ipsilateral axillary lymph nodes
Upper limb:	Ipsilateral epitrochlear and axillary lymph nodes
Abdomen, loins, and buttocks:	Ipsilateral inguinal lymph nodes
Lower limb:	Ipsilateral popliteal and inguinal lymph nodes
Anal margin and perianal skin:	Ipsilateral inguinal lymph nodes

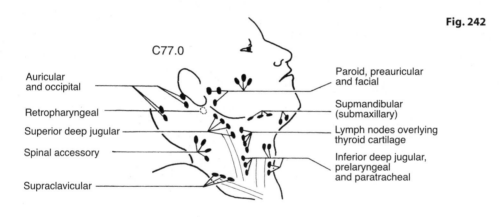

Fig. 242

Skin Tumours

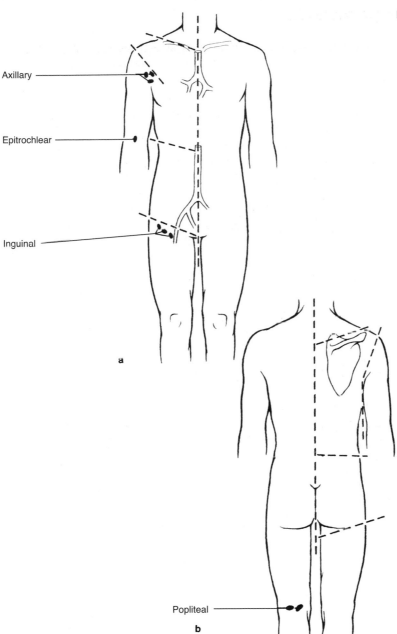

Axillary

Epitrochlear

Inguinal

a

Popliteal

b

Tumours in the Boundary Zones

The lymph nodes pertaining to the regions on both sides of the boundary zone are considered to be the regional lymph nodes. The following 4-cm-wide bands are considered as boundary zones (Figs. 244–248):

Between	Along
Right/left	Midline
Head and neck/thorax	Clavicula–acromion–upper shoulder blade edge
Thorax/upper limb	Shoulder–axilla–shoulder
Thorax/abdomen, loins, and buttocks	*Front:* middle between navel and costal arch *Back:* lower border of thoracic vertebrae (midtransverse axis)
Abdomen, loins, and buttock/lower limb	Groin–trochanter–gluteal sulcus

Any metastasis to other than the listed regional lymph nodes is considered as M1 (Figs. 244–248).

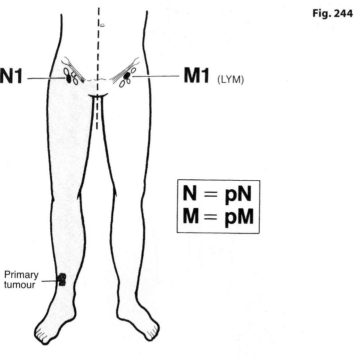

Fig. 244

N1 ——— M1 (LYM)

N = pN
M = pM

Primary tumour

Fig. 245

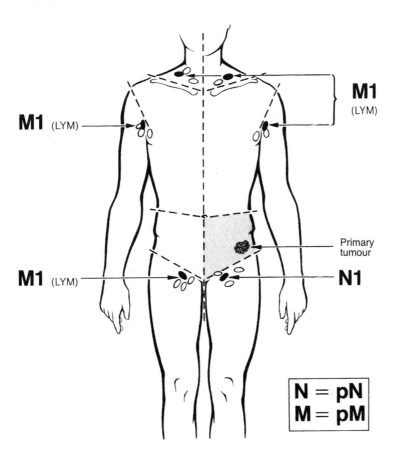

M1 (LYM)

M1 (LYM)

M1 (LYM)

M1 (LYM)

Primary tumour

N1

N = pN
M = pM

Fig. 246

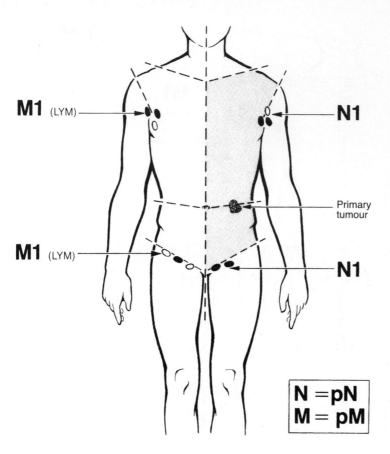

Fig. 247

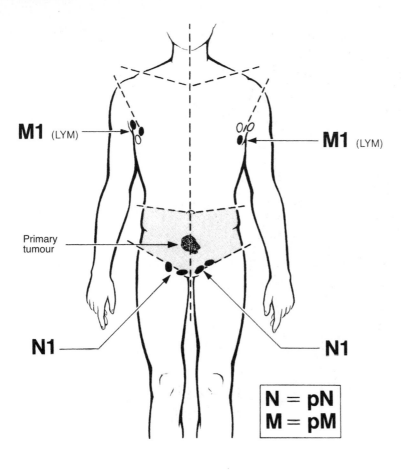

M1 (LYM)

M1 (LYM)

Primary
tumour

N1

N1

N = pN
M = pM

Fig. 248

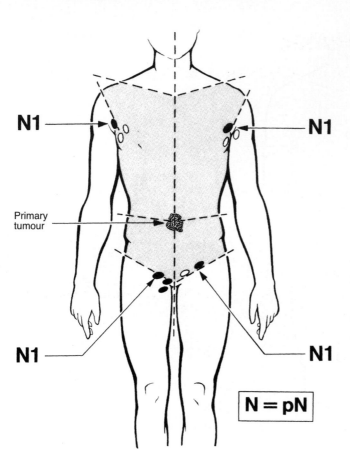

N1

N1

Primary
tumour

N1

N1

N = pN

Carcinoma of the Skin

(excluding eyelid, vulva, and penis) (ICD-O C44.0, 2–9, C63.2)

Rules for Classification

The classification applies only to carcinomas. There should be histological confirmation of the disease and division of cases by histological type.

Regional Lymph Nodes

The regional lymph nodes are those appropriate to the site of the primary tumour. (See p. 184)

TNM Clinical Classification

T – Primary Tumour

TX   Primary tumour cannot be assessed
T0   No evidence of primary tumour
Tis   Carcinoma in situ (Fig. 249)

Tis   pTis   Fig. 249

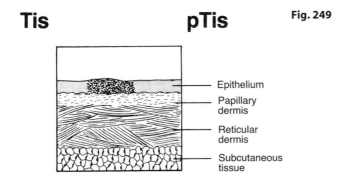

- Epithelium
- Papillary dermis
- Reticular dermis
- Subcutaneous tissue

T1   Tumour 2 cm or less in greatest dimension (Fig. 250)
T2   Tumour more than 2 cm but not more than 5 cm in greatest dimension (Fig. 251)
T3   Tumour more than 5 cm in greatest dimension (Fig. 252)

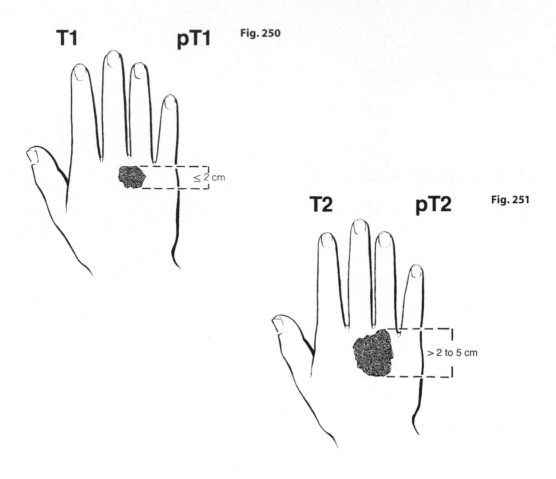

Fig. 250

Fig. 251

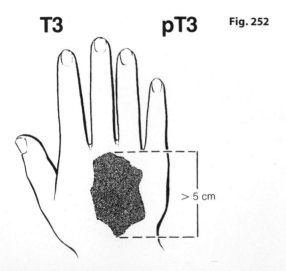

Fig. 252

T4   Tumour invades deep extradermal structures, i.e., cartilage, skeletal muscle, or bone (Fig. 253)

Note
In the case of multiple simultaneous tumours, the tumour with the highest T category is classified and the number of separate tumours is indicated in parentheses, e.g., T2(5) (Fig. 254)

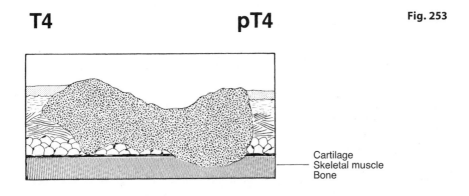

T4   **pT4**   **Fig. 253**

Cartilage
Skeletal muscle
Bone

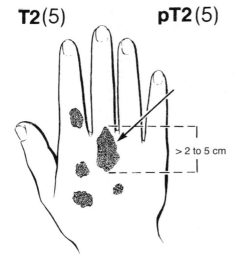

T2(5)   **pT2**(5)   **Fig. 254**

> 2 to 5 cm

N – Regional Lymph Nodes

NX   Regional lymph nodes cannot be assessed
N0   No regional lymph node metastasis
N1   Regional lymph node metastasis (Figs. 244–248, pp. 186–190)

M – Distant Metastasis

MX   Distant metastasis cannot be assessed
M0   No distant metastasis
M1   Distant metastasis (Figs. 244–248, pp. 186–190)

pTNM Pathological Classification

The pT, pN, and pM categories correspond to the T, N, and M categories.

pN0 Histological examination of a regional lymphadenectomy specimen will ordinarily include 6 or more lymph nodes. If the examined lymph nodes are negative, but the number ordinarily resected is not met, classify as pN0.

Malignant Melanoma of Skin

(ICD-O C44, C51.0, C60.9, C63.2)

Rules for Classification

There should be histological confirmation of the disease.

Regional Lymph Nodes

The regional lymph nodes are those appropriate to the site of the primary tumour. (See p. 184)

TNM Clinical Classification

T – Primary Tumour

The extent of the tumour is classified after excision, see pT, p. 204–206

N – Regional Lymph Nodes

NX Regional lymph nodes cannot be assessed
N0 No regional lymph node metastasis

N1 Metastasis in one regional lymph node
N1a Only microscopic metastasis (clinically occult) (Fig. 255)
N1b Macroscopic metastasis (clinically apparent) (Fig. 256)
N2 Metastasis in two or three regional lymph nodes or satellites or in-transit metastasis
N2a Only microscopic metastasis (Fig. 257)
N2b Macroscopic metastasis (Fig. 258)
N2c Satellite ot in-transit metastasis *without* regional lymph node metastasis (Figs. 259, 260)
N3 Metastasis in four or more regional lymph nodes (Fig. 261), or matted metastatic regional lymph nodes (Fig. 262), or satellite(s) or in-transit metastasis with metastasis in regional lymph node(s) (Figs. 263, 264)

Note
Satellites are tumour nests or nodules (macroscopic or microscopic) within 2 cm of the primary tumour. In-transit metastasis involves skin or subcutaneous tissue more than 2 cm from the primary tumour but not beyond the regional lymph nodes.

Malignant Melanoma of Skin

pN1a   Fig. 255

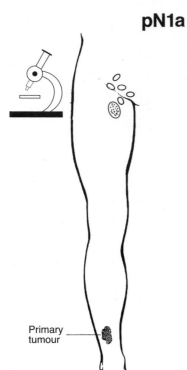

Primary
tumour

N1b   pN1b   Fig. 256

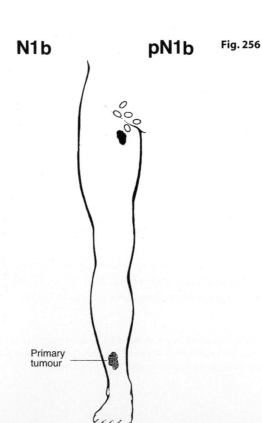

Primary
tumour

pN2a

Fig. 257

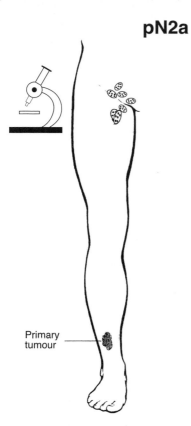

Primary
tumour

N2b   pN2b

Fig. 258

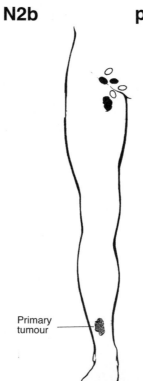

Primary
tumour

N2c   pN2c   Fig. 259

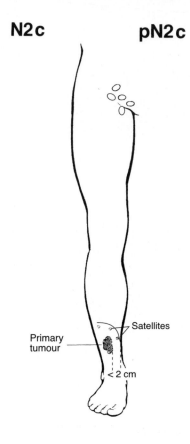

Satellites

Primary
tumour

< 2 cm

N2c   pN2c   Fig. 260

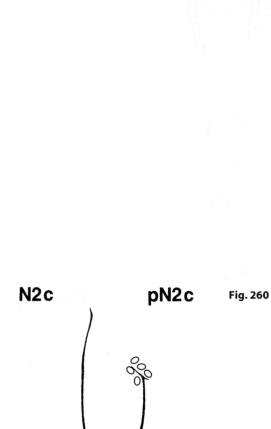

In-transit-
metastasis

Primary
tumour

N3   **pN3**   Fig. 261

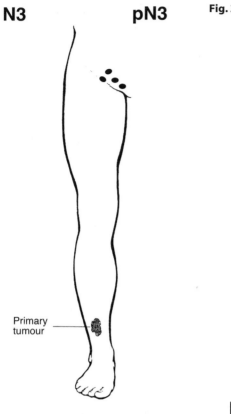

Primary
tumour

N3   **pN3**   Fig. 262

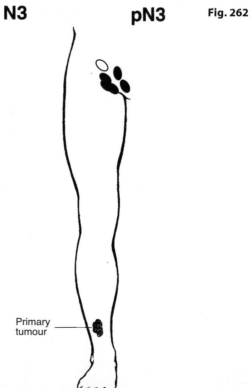

Primary
tumour

N3   **pN3**   **Fig. 263**

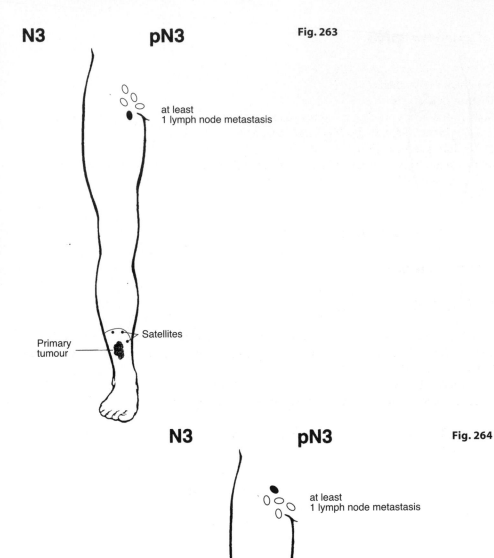

at least
1 lymph node metastasis

Satellites

Primary
tumour

N3   **pN3**   **Fig. 264**

at least
1 lymph node metastasis

In-transit
metastasis

Primary
tumour

M – Distant Metastasis

MX   Distant metastasis cannot be assessed
M0   No distant metastasis
M1   Distant metastasis
      M1a   Metastasis in skin or subcutaneous tissue or lymph node(s) beyond the re-gional lymph nodes (Figs. 244–247, pp. 186–189)
      M1b   Lung metastasis
      M1c   Metastasis in other sites, or any site and an elevated serum lactate dehydroge-nase (LDH)

pTNM Pathological Classification

pT – Primary Tumour

Introductory Note

The pT classification of malignant melanoma considers three histological criteria:
1. Tumour thickness (Breslow) according to the largest vertical diameter of the tumour in millimeters (Fig. 265)
2. Clark "levels" (Fig. 266)
3. Absence or presence of ulceration of the primary tumour (Fig. 265)

The definitive pT category is based on these three criteria.

Malignant Melanoma of Skin

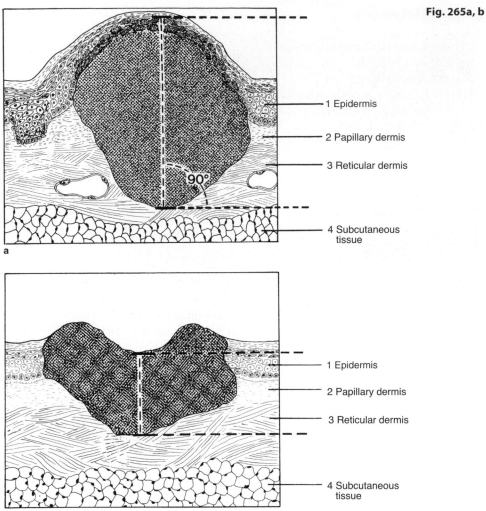

Fig. 265a, b

1 Epidermis

2 Papillary dermis

3 Reticular dermis

4 Subcutaneous tissue

1 Epidermis

2 Papillary dermis

3 Reticular dermis

4 Subcutaneous tissue

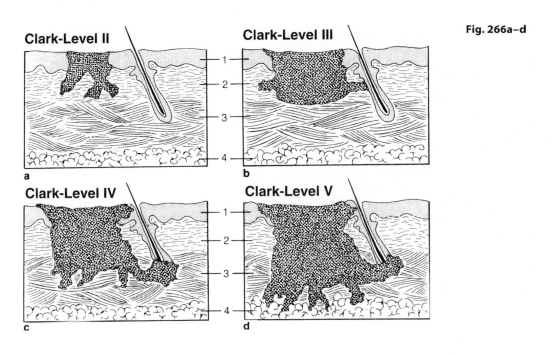

Fig. 266a–d

Clark-Level II

a

Clark-Level III

b

Clark-Level IV

c

Clark-Level V

d

pT – Primary Tumour

pTX   Primary tumour cannot be assessed*
pT0   No evidence of primary tumour
pTis   Melanoma in situ (Clark level I) (atypical melanocytic hyperplasia, severe melanocytic dysplasia, not an invasive malignant lesion)

Note
pTX includes shave biopsies and regressed melanomas.

pT1   Tumour 1 mm or less in thickness (Fig. 267)
    pT1a   Clark level II or III, without ulceration
    pT1b   Clark level IV or V, or with ulceration
pT2   Tumour more than 1 mm but not more than 2 mm in thickness (Fig. 268)
    pT2a   Without ulceration
    pT2b   With ulceration
pT3   Tumour more than 2 mm but not more than 4 mm in thickness (Fig. 269)
    pT3a   Without ulceration
    pT3b   With ulceration

pT1a   pT1b   Fig. 267

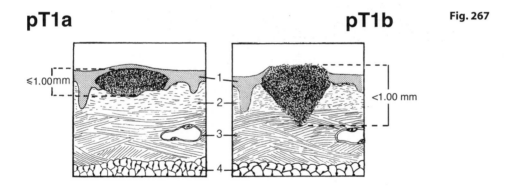

≤1.00mm   1
2
<1.00 mm
3
4

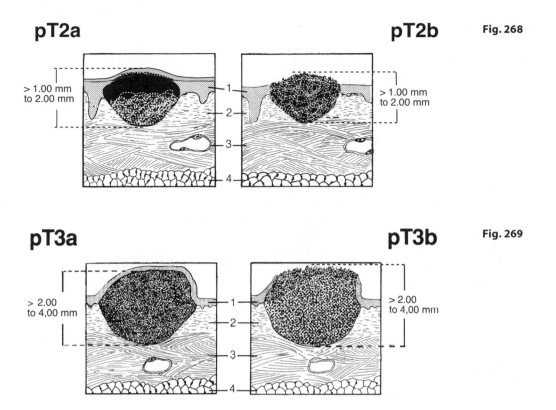

pT2a   pT2b   **Fig. 268**

> 1.00 mm to 2.00 mm

> 1.00 mm to 2.00 mm

pT3a   pT3b   **Fig. 269**

> 2.00 to 4,00 mm

> 2.00 to 4,00 mm

pT4   Tumour more than 4 mm in thickness (Fig. 270)
    pT4a   Without ulceration
    pT4b   With ulceration

pT4a   pT4b

Fig. 270

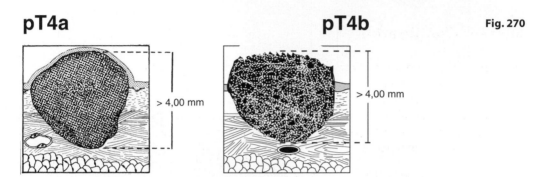

> 4,00 mm

> 4,00 mm

pN – Regional Lymph Nodes

The pN categories correspond to the N categories (see Figs. 255–264, pp. 196–200).

pN0 Histological examination of a regional lymphadenectomy specimen will ordinarily include 6 or more lymph nodes. If the examined lymph nodes are negative, but the number ordinarily resected is not met, classify as pN0. Classification based solely on sentinel lymph node biopsy without subsequent axillary lymph node dissection is designated (sn) for sentinel lymph node, e.g., pN1(sn).

Breast Tumours (ICD-O C50)

Rules for Classification

The classification applies to carcinomas of the male as well as of the female breast. There should be histological confirmation of the disease. The anatomical subsite of origin should be recorded but is not considered in classification.

In the case of multiple simultaneous primary tumours in one breast, the tumour with the highest T category should be used for classification. Simultaneous *bilateral* breast cancers should be classified independently to permit division of cases by histological type.

Anatomical Subsites (Fig. 271)

1. Nipple (C50.0)
2. Central portion (C50.1)
3. Upper-inner quadrant (C50.2)
4. Lower-inner quadrant (C50.3)
5. Upper-outer quadrant (C50.4)
6. Lower-outer quadrant (C50.5)
7. Axillary tail (C50.6)
8. Overlapping lesions (C50.8)

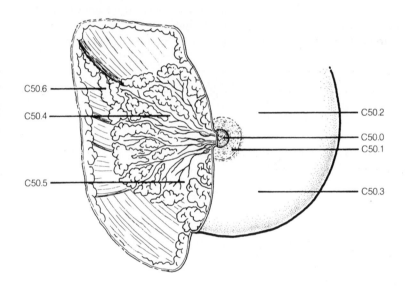

Fig. 271

Regional Lymph Nodes (Fig. 272)

The regional lymph nodes are:

1. *Axillary* (ipsilateral): interpectoral (Rotter) nodes and lymph nodes along the axillary vein and its tributaries, which may be divided into the following levels:
   (i) *Level I* (low-axilla): lymph nodes lateral to the lateral border of pectoralis minor muscle.
   (ii) *Level II* (mid-axilla): lymph nodes between the medial and lateral borders of the pectoralis minor muscle and the interpectoral (Rotter) lymph nodes.
   (iii) *Level III* (apical axilla): apical lymph nodes those medial to the medial margin of the pectoralis minor muscle, excluding those designated as subclavicular or infraclavicular.

Note
Intramammary lymph nodes are coded as axillary lymph nodes.

2. *Infraclavicular* (subclavicular) (ipsilateral).
3. *Internal mammary* (ipsilateral): lymph nodes in the intercostal spaces along the edge of the sternum in the endothoratic fascia.
4. *Supraclavicular* (ipsilateral).

Any other lymph node metastasis is coded as a distant metastasis (M1), including cervical or contralateral internal mammary lymph nodes.

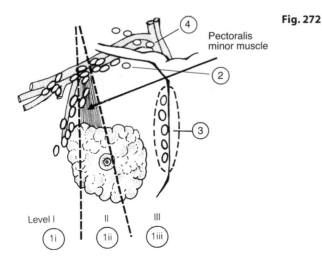

Fig. 272

Pectoralis
minor muscle

TNM Clinical Classification

T – Primary Tumour

TX   Primary tumour cannot be assessed
T0   No evidence of primary tumour
Tis   Carcinoma in situ

Tis (DCIS)   Ductal carcinoma in situ
Tis (LCIS)   Lobular carcinoma in situ
Tis (Paget)   Paget disease of the nipple with no tumour (Fig. 273)

Note
Paget disease associated with a tumour is classified according to the size of the tumour.

T1   Tumour 2 cm or less in greatest dimension
      T1mic   Microinvasion 0.1 cm or less in greatest dimension[1](Fig. 274)
      T1a   More than 0.1 cm but not more than 0.5 cm in greatest dimension (Fig. 275)
      T1b   More than 0.5 cm but not more than 1 cm in greatest dimension (Fig. 275)
      T1c   More than 1 cm but not more than 2 cm in greatest dimension (Fig. 275)
T2   Tumour more than 2 cm but not more than 5 cm in greatest dimension (Fig. 276)

Note
[1] Microinvasion is the extension of cancer cells beyond the basement membrane into the adjacent tissue with no focus more than 0.1 cm in greatest dimension. When there are multiple foci of microinvasion, the size of only the largest focus is used to classify the microinvasion. (Do not use the sum of all individual foci.) The presence of multiple foci of microinvasion should be noted, as it is with multiple larger invasive carcinomas.

Tis

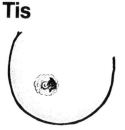

pTis

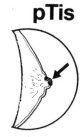

Fig. 273

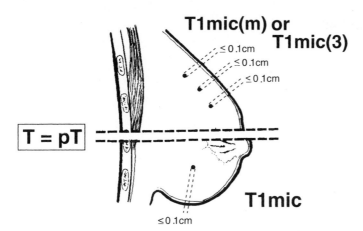

T1mic(m) or T1mic(3)

≤ 0.1cm
≤ 0.1cm
≤ 0.1cm

T = pT

T1mic

≤ 0.1cm

Fig. 274

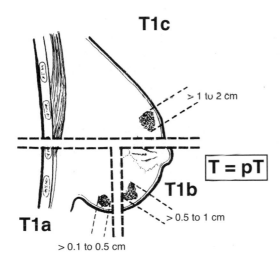

T1c

> 1 to 2 cm

T = pT

T1b

> 0.5 to 1 cm

T1a

> 0.1 to 0.5 cm

Fig. 275

T3   Tumour more than 5 cm in greatest dimension (Fig. 276)

Fig. 276

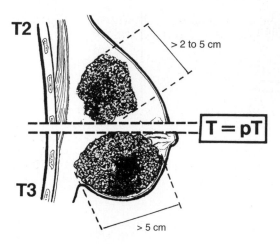

T2

> 2 to 5 cm

T = pT

T3

> 5 cm

T4   Tumour of any size with direct extension to chest wall or skin only as described in T4a to T4d

     T4a   Extension to chest wall[2] (Fig. 277)

     T4b   Oedema (including peau d'orange), or ulceration of the skin of the breast, or satellite skin nodules confined to the same breast (Figs. 278, 279)

     T4c   Both 4a and 4b, above (Fig. 280)

     T4d   Inflammatory carcinoma[3] (Fig. 281)

Note

[2] Chest wall includes ribs, intercostal muscles, and serratus anterior muscle but not pectoral muscle.

[3] Inflammatory carcinoma of the breast is characterized by diffuse, brawny induration of the skin with an erysipeloid edge, usually with no underlying mass. If the skin biopsy is negative and there is no localized measurable primary cancer, the T category is pTX when pathologically staging a clinical inflammatory carcinoma (T4d). Dimpling of the skin, nipple retraction, or other skin changes, except those in T4b and T4d, may occur in T1, T2, or T3 without affecting the classification.

T4a   **pT4a**   **Fig. 277**

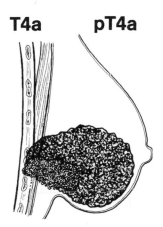

T4b   **pT4b**   **Fig. 278**

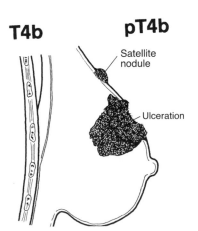

Satellite nodule

Ulceration

T4b   pT4b

Fig. 279

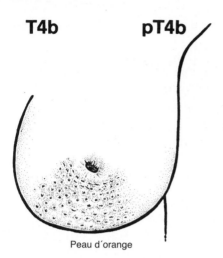

Peau d´orange

T4c   pT4c

Fig. 280

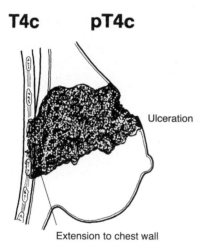

Ulceration

Extension to chest wall

T4d   pT4d

Fig. 281

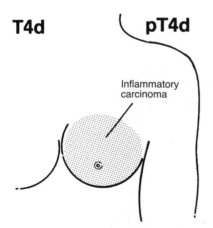

Inflammatory
carcinoma

N – Regional Lymph Nodes

NX   Regional lymph nodes cannot be assessed (e.g., previously removed)

N0   No regional lymph node metastasis

N1   Metastasis in movable ipsilateral axillary node(s) (Fig. 282)

N2   Metastasis in fixed ipsilateral axillary lymph node(s) or in clinically apparent* ipsilateral internal mammary lymph node(s) in the absence of clinically evident axillary lymph node metastasis

        N2a   Metastasis in ipsilateral axillary lymph node(s) fixed to one another or to other structures (Fig. 283)

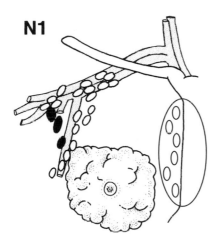

N1

Fig. 282

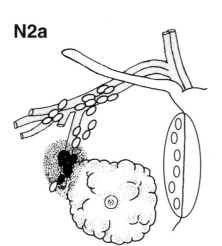

N2a

Fig. 283

N2b   Metastasis only in clinically apparent* ipsilateral internal mammary lymph node(s) and in the absence of clinically evident ipsilateral axillary lymph node metastasis (Fig. 284)

N3   Metastasis into ipsilateral infraclavicular lymph node(s) with or without axillary lymph node(s); or in clinically apparent* ipsilateral internal mammary lymph node(s) and when occuring in the presence of clinically evident axillary lymph node metastasis; or metastasis in ipsilateral supraclavicular lymph node(s) with or without axillary or internal mammary lymph node involvement

N2b

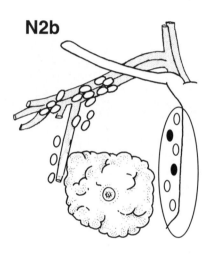

Fig. 284

N3a

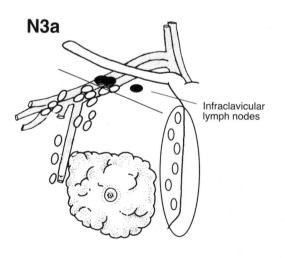

Fig. 285

Infraclavicular lymph nodes

Breast Tumours

N3a Metastasis in ipsilateral infraclavicular lymph node(s) (Fig. 285)
N3b Metastasis in ipsilateral internal mammary and axillary lymph nodes (Fig. 286)
N3c Metastasis in ipsilateral supraclavicular lymph node(s) (Fig. 287)

Note
* Clinically apparent = detected by imaging studies (excluding lymphscintigraphy) or by clinical examination

Fig. 286

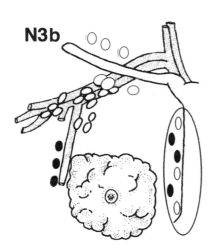

Fig. 287

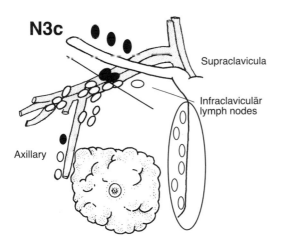

pTNM Pathological Classification

pT – Primary Tumour

The pathological classification requires the examination of the primary carcinoma with no gross tumour at the margins of resection. A case can be classified pT if there is only microscopic tumour in a margin.

The pT categories correspond to the T categories.

Note
When classifying pT the tumour size is a measurement of the invasive component. If there is a large in situ component (e.g., 4 cm) and a small invasive component (e.g., 0.5 cm), the tumour is coded pT1a.

pN – Regional Lymph Nodes

The pathological classification requires the resection and examination of at least the low axillary lymph nodes (level I) (see p. 209). Such a resection will ordinarily include 6 or more lymph nodes. If the examined lymph nodes are negative, but the number ordinarily resected is not met, classify as pN0.

Examination of one or more sentinel lymph nodes may be used for pathological classification. If classification is based solely on sentinel lymph node biopsy without subsequent axillary lymph node dissection it should be designated (sn) for sentinel lymph node, e.g., pN1(sn).

pNX   Regional lymph nodes cannot be assessed (not removed for study or previously removed)
pN0   No regional lymph node metastasis

Note

Cases with only isolated tumour cells (ITC) in regional lymph nodes are classified as pN0. ITC are single tumour cells or small clusters of cells, not more than 0.2 mm in greatest dimension, that are usually detected by immunohistochemistry or molecular methods but which may be verified on H&E stains. ITC do not typically show evidence of metastatic activity, e.g., proliferation or stromal reaction.

pN1(mi) Micrometastasis (greater than 0.2 mm but not more than 2.0 mm in greatest dimension) (Fig. 288)

pN1 Metastasis in 1 to 3 ipsilateral axillary lymph node(s), and/ or in ipsilateral internal mammary lymph nodes with microscopic metastasis detected by sentinel lymph node dissection but not clinically apparent**

  pN1a Metastasis in 1 to 3 axillary lymph node(s), including at least one larger than 2.0 mm in greatest dimension (Fig. 289)

pN1 mi

Fig. 288

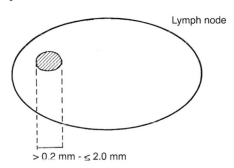

Lymph node

> 0.2 mm - ≤ 2.0 mm

pN1a

Fig. 289

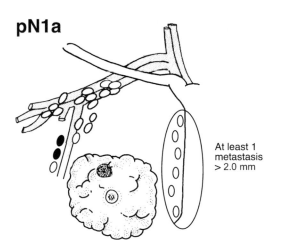

At least 1 metastasis > 2.0 mm

pN1b   Internal mammary lymph nodes with microscopic metastasis detected by
       sentinel lymph node dissection but not clinically apparent** (Fig. 290)
pN1c   Metastasis in 1 to 3 axillary lymph nodes and in internal mammary lymph
       nodes with microscopic metastasis detected by sentinel lymph node dissec-
       tion but not clinically apparent** (Fig. 291)

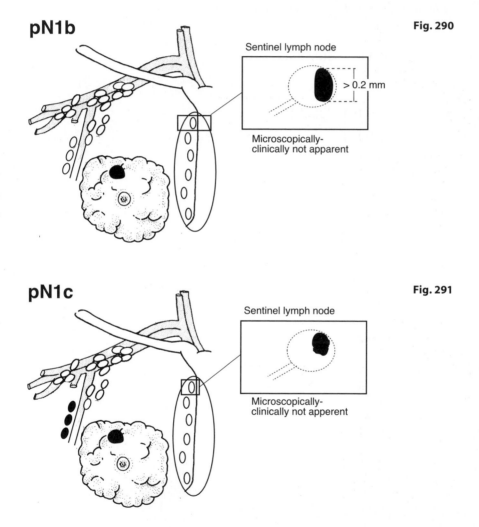

pN1b

Fig. 290

Sentinel lymph node

> 0.2 mm

Microscopically-
clinically not apparent

pN1c

Fig. 291

Sentinel lymph node

Microscopically-
clinically not apperent

pN2   Metastasis in 4 to 9 ipsilateral axillary lymph nodes, or in clinically apparent** internal mammary lymph node(s) in the absence of axillary lymph node metastasis

     pN2a   Metastasis in 4 to 9 axillary lymph nodes, including at least one that is larger than 2.0 mm in greatest dimension (Fig. 292)

     pN2b   Metastasis in clinically apparent** internal mammary lymph node(s), in the *absence* of axillary lymph node metastasis (Fig. 293)

pN2a

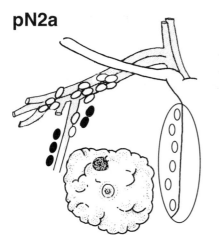

Fig. 292

4 - 9 axillary lymph node
metastases,
at least 1 metastasis
> 2.0 mm

pN2b

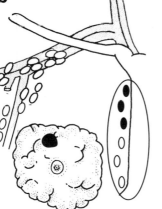

Fig. 293

Internal mammary
lymph nodes,
clinically apparent

pN3   Metastasis in 10 or more ipsilateral axillary lymph nodes; or in ipsilateral infracla-
       vicular lymph nodes; or in clinically apparent** ipsilateral internal mammary lymph
       nodes in the *presence* of one or more positive axillary lymph nodes; or in more than
       3 axillary lymph nodes with clinically negative, microscopic metastasis in internal
       mammary lymph nodes; or in ipsilateral supraclavicular lymph nodes
       pN3a Metastasis in 10 or more axillary lymph nodes (at least one larger than 2 mm
             in greatest dimension) or metastasis in infraclavicular lymph nodes (Figs. 294,
             295)

pN3a

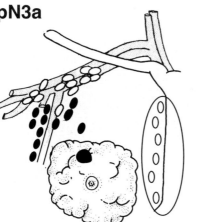

Fig. 294

≥ 10 axillary lymph node metastasis,
at least one metastasis > 0.2 cm

pN3a

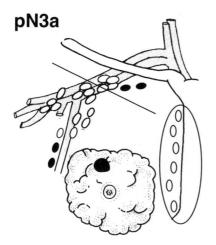

Fig. 295

pN3b   Metastasis in clinically apparent** internal mammary lymph node(s) in the *presence* of one or more positive axillary lymph node(s) (Fig. 296); or metastasis in more than 3 axillary lymph nodes *and* in internal mammary lymph nodes with microscopic metastasis detected by sentinel lymph node dissection but not clinically apparent*

pN3c   Metastasis in supraclavicular lymph nodes (Fig. 297)

Note

*   Not clinically apparent = not detected by clinical examination or by imaging studies (excluding lymphoscintigraphy)

** Clinically apparent: detected by clinical examination or by imaging studies (excluding lymphoscintigraphy) or grossly visible pathologically.

pN3b

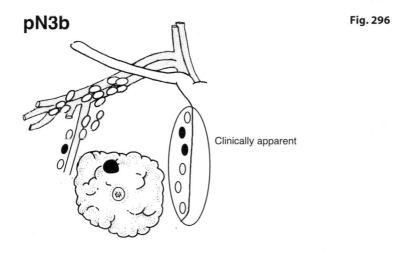

Fig. 296

Clinically apparent

pN3c

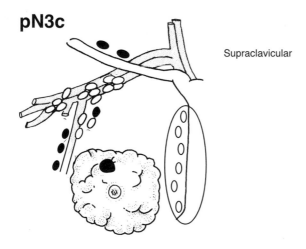

Fig. 297

Supraclavicular

pM – Distant Metastasis

The pM categories correspond to the M categories.

Gynaecological Tumours

Introductory Notes

The following sites are included:

- Vulva
- Vagina
- Cervix uteri
- Corpus uteri
- Ovary
- Fallopian tube
- Gestational trophoblastic tumours

Cervix uteri and corpus uteri were among the first sites to be classified by the TNM system. The "League of Nations" stages for carcinoma of the cervix have been used with minor modifications for over 50 years, and, because these are accepted by the Fédération Internationale de Gynécologie et d'Obstétrique (FIGO), the TNM categories have been defined to correspond to the FIGO stages. Some amendments have been made in collaboration with FIGO, and the classifications now published have the approval of the FIGO, UICC, and the national TNM committees including the AJCC.

Vulva (ICD-O C51)

The definitions of the T, N, and M categories correspond to FIGO stages. Both systems are included for comparison.

Rules for Classification

The classification applies only to primary carcinomas of the vulva. There should be histological confirmation of the disease.

A carcinoma of the vulva that has extended to the vagina is classified as carcinoma of the vulva.

The FIGO stages are based on surgical staging. TNM stages are based on clinical and/or pathological classification.

Anatomical Subsites (Fig. 298)

1. Labia majora (C51.0)
2. Labia minora (C51.1)
3. Clitoris (C51.2)

Regional Lymph Nodes

The regional lymph nodes are the femoral and inguinal nodes.

Vulva

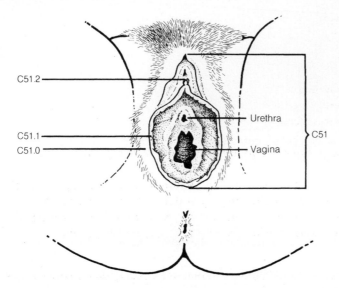

Fig. 298

C51.2

C51.1

C51.0

Urethra

Vagina

C51

TN Clinical Classification

T – Primary Tumour

TX   Primary tumour cannot be assessed

T0   No evidence of primary tumour

Tis   Carcinoma in situ (preinvasive carcinoma)

T1   Tumour confined to vulva or vulva and perineum, 2 cm or less in greatest dimension (Fig. 299)

    T1a   Tumour confined to vulva or vulva and perineum, 2 cm or less in greatest dimension and with stromal invasion no greater than 1.0 mm* (Fig. 300a)

    T1b   Tumour confined to vulva or vulva and perineum, 2 cm or less in greatest dimension and with stromal invasion greater than 1.0 mm* (Fig. 300b)

Note

* The depth of invasion is defined as the measurement of the tumour from the epithelial-stromal junction of the adjacent most superficial dermal papilla to the deepest point of invasion.

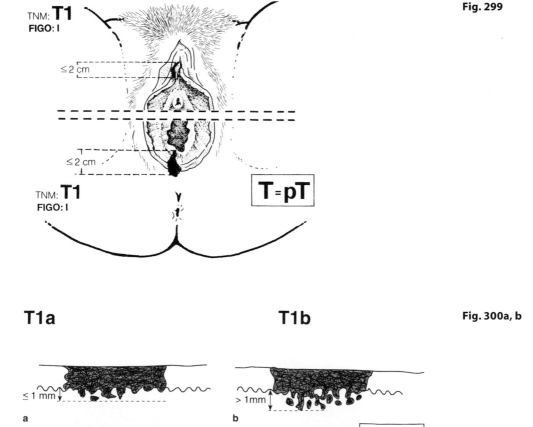

Fig. 299

TNM: **T1**
FIGO: I

≤ 2 cm

≤ 2 cm

TNM: **T1**
FIGO: I

T = pT

T1a

T1b

Fig. 300a, b

≤ 1 mm

> 1mm

a

b

T = pT

Vulva

T2   Tumour confined to vulva or vulva and perineum, more than 2 cm in greatest dimension (Fig. 301)
T3   Tumour invades any of the following: lower urethra, vagina, anus (Figs. 302, 303)

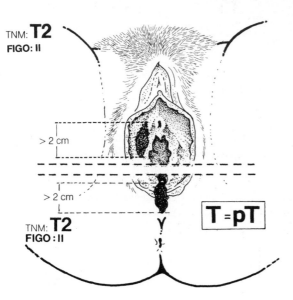

Fig. 301

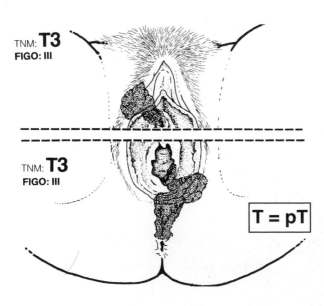

Fig. 302

T4   Tumour invades any of the following: bladder mucosa, rectal mucosa, upper urethral mucosa; or is fixed to pubic bone (Fig. 304)

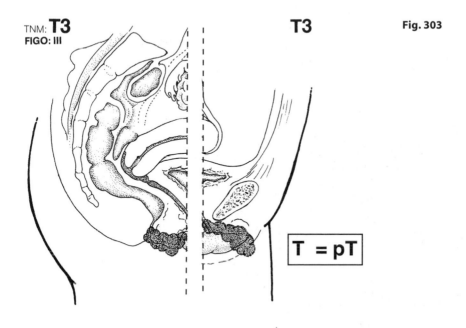

TNM: **T3**
FIGO: III

T3

Fig. 303

T = pT

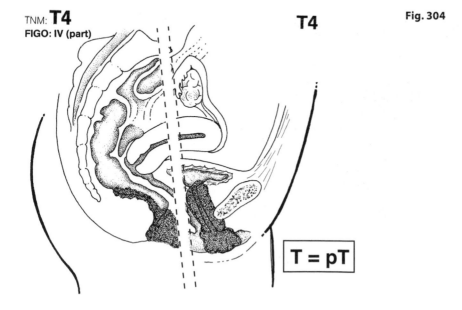

TNM: **T4**
FIGO: IV (part)

T4

Fig. 304

T = pT

N – Regional Lymph Nodes

NX   Regional lymph nodes cannot be assessed
N0   No regional lymph node metastasis
N1   Unilateral regional lymph node metastasis (Fig. 305)
N2   Bilateral regional lymph node metastasis (Fig. 306)

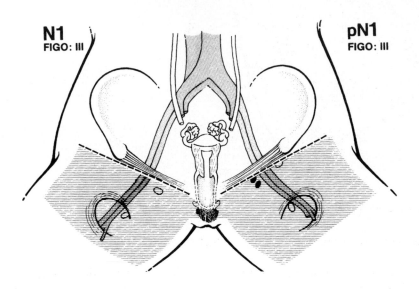

N1
FIGO: III

pN1
FIGO: III

Fig. 305

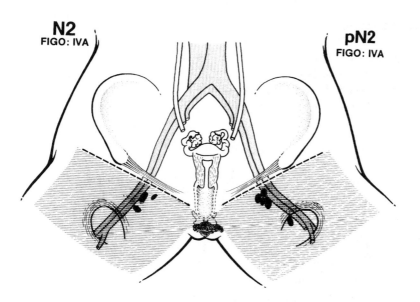

N2
FIGO: IVA

pN2
FIGO: IVA

Fig. 306

pTN Pathological Classification

The pT and pN categories correspond to the T and N categories.

pN0 Histological examination of an inguinal lymphadenectomy specimen will ordinarily include 6 or more lymph nodes.

If the examined lymph nodes are negative, but the number ordinarily resected is not met, classify as pN0.

Vagina (ICD-O C52) (Fig. 307)

The definitions of the T and M categories correspond to the FIGO stages. Both systems are included for comparison.

The FIGO stages are based on clinical staging. (TNM stages are based on clinical and/or pathological classification).

Rules for Classification

The classification applies to primary carcinomas only.

Tumours present in the vagina as secondary growths from either genital or extragenital sites are excluded.

A tumour that has extended to the portio and reached the external os (orifice of uterus) is classified as carcinoma of the cervix.

A tumour involving the vulva is classified as carcinoma of the vulva.

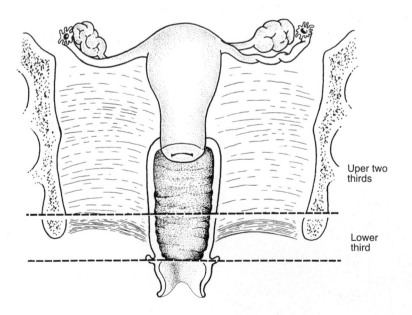

Fig. 307

Uper two
thirds

Lower
third

Regional Lymph Nodes

Upper two-thirds of vagina:
The pelvic nodes including obturator, internal iliac (hypogastric), external iliac, and pelvic nodes, NOS (Fig. 308).

Lower third of vagina:
The inguinal nodes and femoral nodes (Fig. 309).

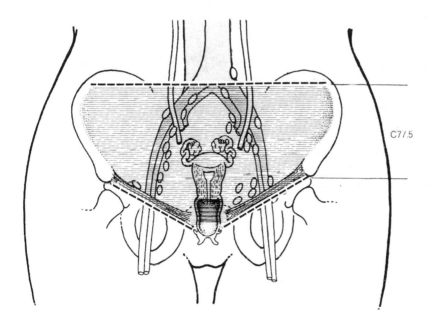

Fig. 308

C7/.5

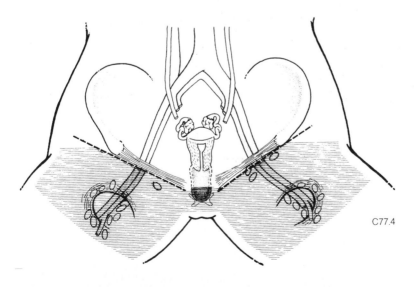

Fig. 309

C77.4

TNM Clinical Classification

T – Primary Tumour

TNM categories	FIGO stages	
TX		Primary tumour cannot be assessed
T0		No evidence of primary tumour
Tis		Carcinoma in situ (preinvasive carcinoma)
T1	I	Tumour confined to vagina (Fig. 310)
T2	II	Tumour invades paravaginal tissues but does not extend to pelvic wall (Fig. 311)
T3	III	Tumour extends to pelvic wall (Fig. 312)
T4	IVA	Tumour invades mucosa of the bladder or rectum and/or extends beyond the true pelvis (Fig. 313)

Note
The presence of bullous oedema is not sufficient evidence to classify a tumour as T4.

Vagina

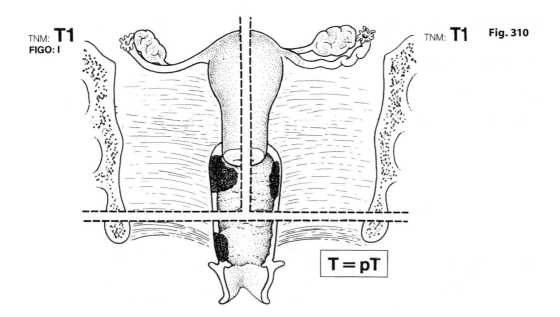

TNM: **T1**
FIGO: I

TNM: **T1**   Fig. 310

T = pT

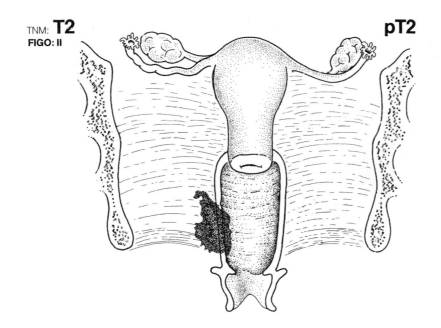

TNM: **T2**
FIGO: II

pT2   Fig. 311

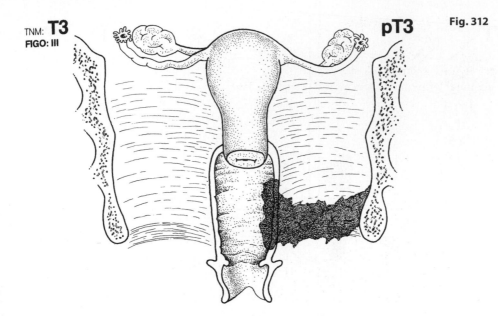

TNM: **T3**
FIGO: III

pT3

Fig. 312

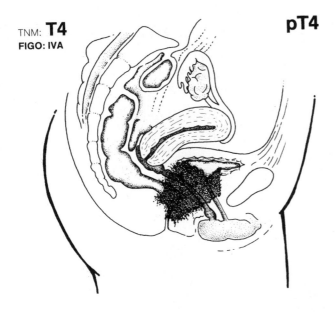

TNM: **T4**
FIGO: IVA

pT4

Fig. 313

N – Regional Lymph Nodes

NX   Regional lymph nodes cannot be assessed
N0   No regional lymph node metastasis
N1   Regional lymph node metastasis (Figs. 314–316)

N1   **pN1**

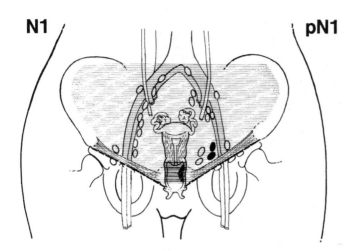

Fig. 314

N1

pN1

Fig. 315

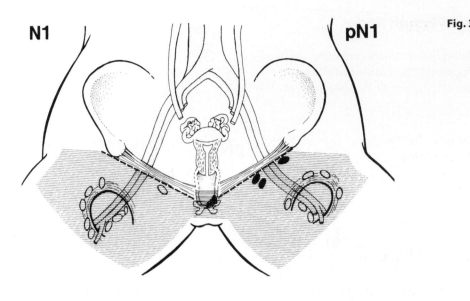

N1

pN1

Fig. 316

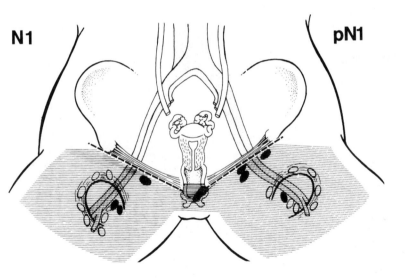

pTN Pathological Classification

The pT and pN categories correspond to the T and N categories.

pN0 Histological examination of an inguinal lymphadenectomy specimen will ordinarily include 6 or more lymph nodes; a pelvic lymphadenectomy specimen will ordinarily include 10 or more lymph nodes.

If the examined lymph nodes are negative, but the number ordinarily resected is not met, classify as pN0.

Cervix Uteri (ICD-O C53)

The definitions of the T and M categories correspond to the FIGO stages. Both systems are included for comparison.

The FIGO stages are based on clinical staging. This includes histological examination of a cone or amputation of the cervix. (TNM stages are based on clinical and/or pathological classification.)

Rules for Classification

The classification applies only to carcinomas. There should be histological confirmation of the disease.

Anatomical Subsites (Fig. 317)

1. Endocervix (C53.0)
2. Exocervix (C53.1)

Fig. 317

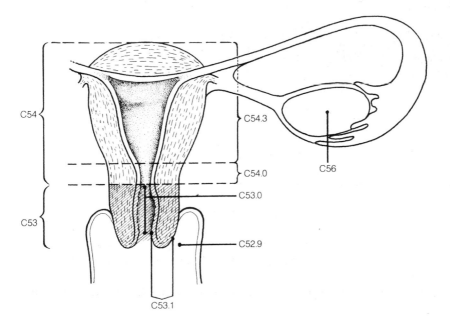

Regional Lymph Nodes (Fig. 318)

The regional lymph nodes are:
(1) paracervical nodes
(2) parametrial nodes
(3) hypogastric (internal iliac) including obturator nodes
(4) external iliac nodes
(5) common iliac nodes
(6) presacral nodes
(7) lateral sacral nodes (not shown in Fig. 318)

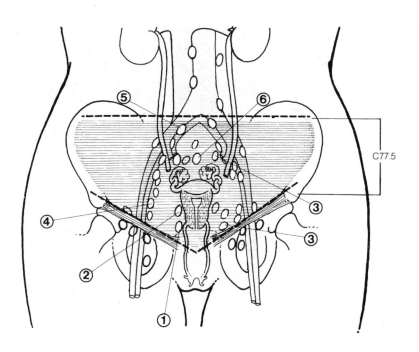

Fig. 318

C77.5

TNM Clinical Classification

T – Primary Tumour

TNM categories	FIGO stages	
TX		Primary tumour cannot be assessed
T0		No evidence of primary
Tis	0	Carcinoma in situ (preinvasive carcinoma)
T1	I	Cervical carcinoma confined to uterus (extension to corpus should be disregarded)
T1a	IA	Invasive carcinoma diagnosed only by microscopy. All macroscopically visible lesions–even with superficial invasion–are T1b/Stage IB (Fig. 319a-c)
T1a1	IA1	Stromal invasion no greater than 3.0 mm in depth and 7.0 mm or less in horizontal spread (Fig. 320a-c)
T1a2	IA2	Stromal invasion more than 3.0 mm and not more than 5.0 mm with a horizontal spread 7.0 mm or less (Fig. 321a-c)

Note
The depth of invasion should not be more than 5.0 mm taken from the base of the epithelium, either surface or glandular, from which it originates. The depth of invasion is defined as the measurement of the tumour from the epithelial-stromal junction of the adjacent most superficial epithelial papilla to the deepest point of invasion.

TNM categories	FIGO stages	
T1b	IB	Clinically visible lesion confined to the cervix (Figs. 322, 324) or microscopic lesion greater than T1a2/IA2 (Fig. 323)*
T1b1	IB1	Clinically visible lesion 4.0 cm or less in greatest dimension (Fig. 322)
T1b2	IB2	Clinically visible lesion more than 4.0 cm in greatest dimension (Fig. 324)
T2	II	Tumour invades beyond uterus but not to pelvic wall or to lower third of the vagina (Fig. 325)
T2a	IIA	Without parametrial invasion
T2b	IIB	With parametrial invasion

* Note:
Lesions diagnosed only by microscopy greater than T1a2/IA2 should be classified as T1b1/IB1

TNM: **T1a**   **pT1a**

FIGO: IA

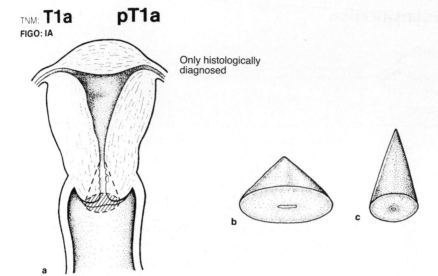

Only histologically
diagnosed

a

b

c

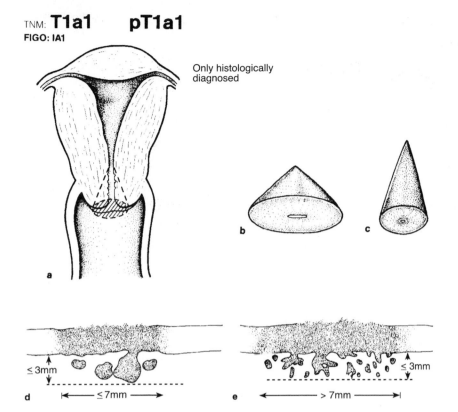

TNM: **T1a1**   **pT1a1**

FIGO: IA1

Only histologically
diagnosed

≤ 3mm

d   ≤ 7mm

≤ 3mm

e   > 7mm

TNM **T1a2**   **pT1a2**
FIGO: IA 2

Fig. 321a-c

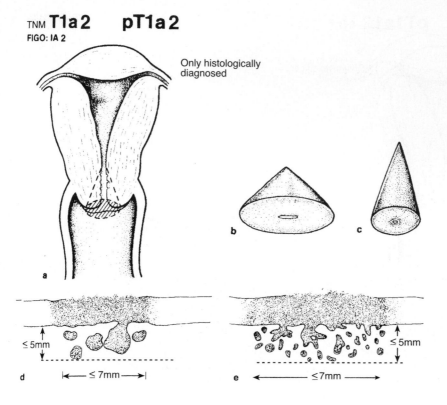

Only histologically
diagnosed

≤ 5mm

d |← ≤ 7mm →|

≤ 5mm

e   ← ≤7mm →

TNM: **T1b1**   **pT1b1**
FIGO:IB1

Fig. 322

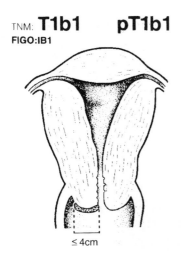

≤ 4cm

TNM: **T1b1**
FIGO: IB1

pT1b1

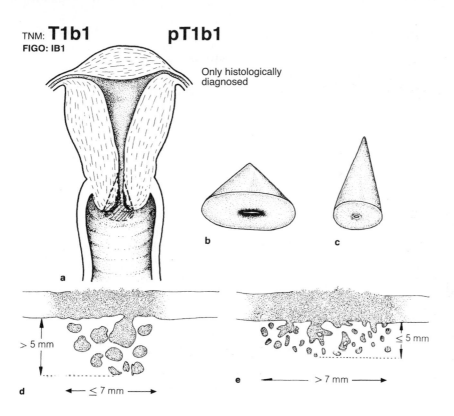

Only histologically
diagnosed

b

c

> 5 mm

≤ 5 mm

d

≤ 7 mm

e

> 7 mm

TNM: **T1b2**
FIGO: IB2

pT1b2

Fig. 324

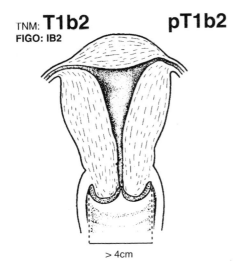

> 4cm

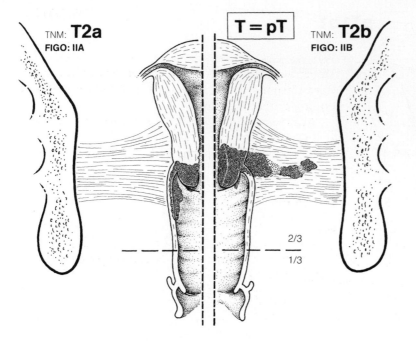

Fig. 325

TNM: **T2a**
FIGO: IIA

T = pT

TNM: **T2b**
FIGO: IIB

2/3
1/3

TNM categories	FIGO stages	
T3	III	Tumour extends to pelvic wall and/or involves the lower third of vagina and/or causes hydrnephrosis or non-functioning kidney (Fig. 326)
T3a	IIIA	Tumour involves lower third of vagina, no extension to pelvic wall
T3b	IIIB	Tumour extends to pelvic wall and/or causes hydronephrosis or non-functioning kidney
T4	IVA	Tumour invades mucosa of bladder or rectum and/or extends beyond true pelvis (Fig. 327)

Note
The presence of bullous oedema is not sufficient evidence to classify a tumour as T4. Invasion of bladder and rectum mucosa should be biopsy proven.

M1	IVB	Distant metastasis

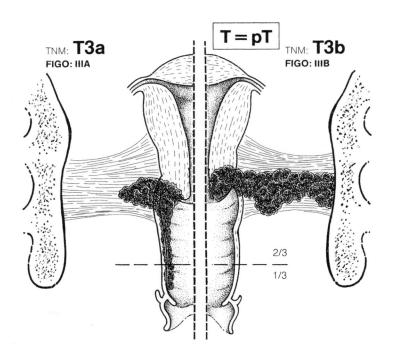

Fig. 326

T = pT

TNM: **T3a**
FIGO: IIIA

TNM: **T3b**
FIGO: IIIB

2/3
1/3

TNM: **T4**
FIGO: IVA

pT4

Fig. 327

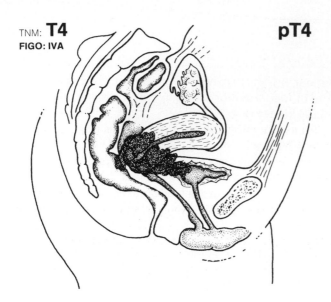

N – Regional Lymph Nodes

NX   Regional lymph nodes cannot be assessed
N0   No regional lymph node metastasis
N1   Regional lymph node metastasis (Fig. 328)

pTNM Pathological Classification

The pT, pN and pM categories correspond to the T, N and pM categories.

pN0 Histological examination of a pelvic lymphadenectomy specimen will ordinarily include 10 or more lymph nodes.
    If the examined lymph nodes are negative, but the number ordinarily resected is not met, classify as pN0.

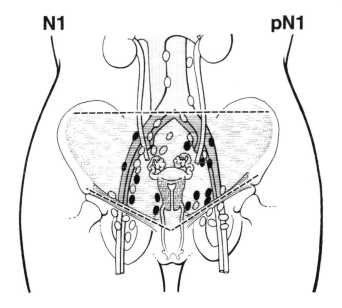

N1   **pN1**   **Fig. 328**

Corpus Uteri (ICD-O C54)

The definitions of the T, N, and M categories correspond to the FIGO stages. Both systems are included for comparison.

The FIGO stages are based on surgical staging. (TNM stages are based on clinical and/or pathological classification).

Rules for Classification

The classification applies only to carcinomas and malignant mixed mesodermal tumours. There should be histological verification with subdivision of histological type and grading of the carcinomas. The diagnosis should be based on examination of specimens taken by endometrial biopsy.

Editors' Note
FIGO does not recommend this classification for mixed mesodermal tumours.

The FIGO recommends for stage I patients who undergo primary a radiotherapy the following clinical classification:

Stage I: Tumour limited to corpus uteri
Stage IA: Length of the uterine cavity 8 cm or less
Stage IB: Length of uterine cavity more than 8 cm

Anatomical Subsites (Fig. 317, p. 239)

1. Isthmus uteri (C54.0)
2. Fundus uteri (C54.3)

Regional Lymph Nodes (Fig. 334, p. 255)

The regional lymph nodes are:
(1) the pelvic lymph nodes
   - hypogastric [obturator, internal iliac (1)]
   - common iliac (2)
   - external iliac (3)
   - parametrial (not shown in figures)
   - sacral (presacral, lateral sacral) (4)
and
(2) the para-aortic lymph nodes including paracaval and interaortocaval lymph nodes (5).

TNM Clinical Classification

T – Primary Tumour

TNM categories	FIGO stages		
TX			Primary tumour cannot be assessed
T0			No evidence of primary tumour
Tis	0		Carcinoma in situ (preinvasive carcinoma)
T1	I		Tumour confined to corpus uteri (Fig. 329)
T1a		IA	Tumour limited to endometrium
T1b		IB	Tumour invades less than one half of myometrium
T1c		IC	Tumour invades one half or more of myometrium
T2	II		Tumour invades cervix but does not extend beyond uterus (Fig. 330)
T2a		IIA	Endocervical glandular involvement only
T2b		IIB	Cervical stromal invasion
T3 and/or N1	III		Local and/or regional spread as specified in T3a, b, N1, and FIGO IIIA, B, C below
T3a		IIIA	Tumour involves serosa and/or adnexa (direct extension or metastasis) and/or cancer cells in ascites or peritoneal washings (Fig. 331)
T3b		IIIB	Vaginal involvement (direct extension or metastasis) (Fig. 331)
N1		IIIC	Metastasis to pelvic and/or para-aortic lymph nodes (Fig. 333)
T4		IVA	Tumour invades bladder *mucosa* and/or bowel *mucosa* (Fig. 332)

Note
The presence of bullous edema is not sufficient evidence to classify a tumour as T4. The lesions should be confirmed by biopsy.

M1		IVB	Distant metastasis (*excluding* metastasis to vagina, pelvic serosa, or adnexa, *including* metastasis to intra-abdominal lymph nodes other than para-aortic, and/or pelvic nodes)

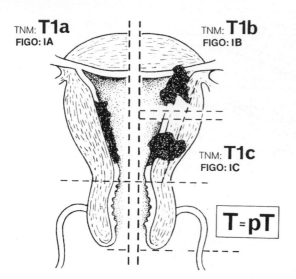

TNM: **T1a**
FIGO: IA

TNM: **T1b**
FIGO: IB

TNM: **T1c**
FIGO: IC

Fig. 329

$$T = pT$$

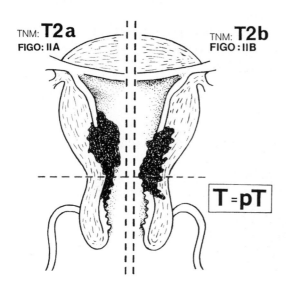

TNM: **T2a**
FIGO: IIA

TNM: **T2b**
FIGO: IIB

Fig. 330

$$T = pT$$

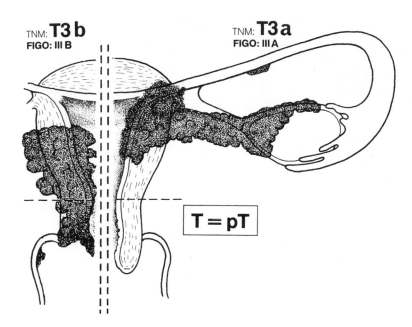

TNM: **T3b**
FIGO: III B

TNM: **T3a**
FIGO: III A

Fig. 331

$$T = pT$$

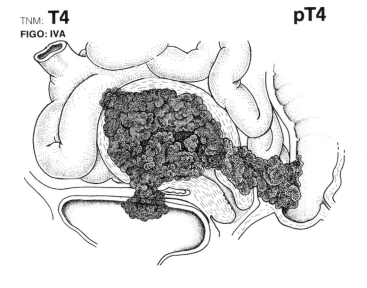

TNM: **T4**
FIGO: IVA

pT4

Fig. 332

N – Regional Lymph Nodes

NX　Regional lymph nodes cannot be assessed
N0　No regional lymph node metastasis
N1　Regional lymph node metastasis (Fig. 333)

pTN Pathological Classification

The pT and pN categories correspond to the T and N   categories.

pN0 Histological examination of a pelvic lymphadenectomy specimen will ordinarily include 10 or more lymph nodes.
　If the examined lymph nodes are negative, but the number ordinarily resected is not met, classify as pN0.

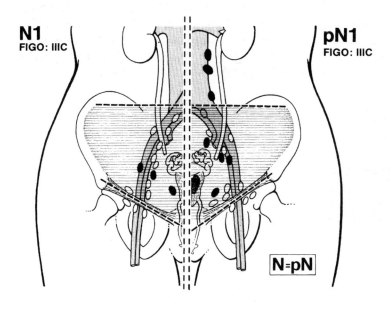

N1
FIGO: IIIC

pN1
FIGO: IIIC

Fig. 333

N=pN

Ovary (ICD-O C56)

The definitions of the T, N, and M categories correspond to the FIGO stages. Both systems are included for comparison.

The FIGO stages are based on clinical staging. (TNM stages are based on clinical and/or pathological classification.)

Rules for Classification

The classification applies to malignant surface epithelial-stromal tumours including those of borderline malignancy or low malignant potential (WHO Classification of Tumours. Pathology and Genetics. Tumours of the Breast and Female Genital Organs. Tavassoli FA, Devilee P, eds., 2003) corresponding to "common epithelial tumours" of earlier terminology. Non-epithelial ovarian cancers may also be classified using this scheme*. There should be histological confirmation of the disease and division of cases by histological type.

Note of editors:
* This possibility is not given in the FIGO classification.

Regional Lymph Nodes (Fig. 334)

The regional lymph nodes are
(1) hypogastric (including obturator)
(2) common iliac
(3) external iliac
(4) lateral sacral
(5) para-aortic
(6) inguinal nodes.

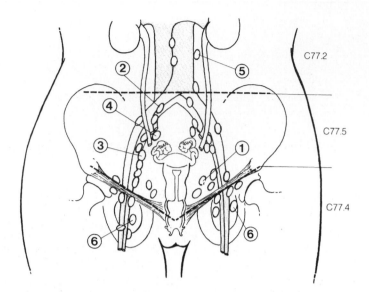

Fig. 334

TNM Clinical Classification

T – Primary Tumour

TNM categories	FIGO stages	
TX		Primary tumour cannot be assessed
T0		No evidence of primary tumour
T1	I	Tumour limited to the ovaries
T1a	IA	Tumour limited to one ovary; capsule intact, no tumour on ovarian surface; no malignant cells in ascites or peritoneal washings (Fig. 335)
T1b	IB	Tumour limited to both ovaries; capsule intact, no tumour on ovarian surface; no malignant cells in ascites or peritoneal washings (Fig. 336)

Ovary

TNM categories	FIGO stages	
T1c	IC	Tumour limited to one or both ovaries with any of the following: capsule ruptured, tumour on ovarian surface, malignant cells in ascites or peritoneal washings* (Fig. 337)
T2	II	Tumour involves one or both ovaries with pelvic extension
T2a	IIA	Extension and/or implants on uterus and/or tube(s) (Fig. 338); no malignant cells in ascites or peritoneal washings
T2b	IIB	Extension to other pelvic tissues; no malignant cells in ascites or peritoneal washings* (Fig. 339)
T2c	IIC	Pelvic extension (2a or 2b) with malignant cells in ascites or peritoneal washings* (Fig. 340)
T3 and/ or N1	III	Tumour involves one or both ovaries with microscopically confirmed peritoneal metastasis outside the pelvis and/ or regional lymph node metastasis (Figs. 341–343)
T3a	IIIA	Microscopic peritoneal metastasis beyond pelvis
T3b	IIIB	Macroscopic peritoneal metastasis beyond pelvis 2 cm or less in greatest dimension
T3c and/ or N1	IIIC	Peritoneal metastasis beyond pelvis more than 2 cm in greatest dimension and/or regional lymph node metastasis (Fig. 343)
M1	IV	Distant metastasis (excludes peritoneal metastasis) (Fig. 342)

Note

Liver capsule metastasis is T3/stage III, liver parenchymal metastasis M1/stage IV. Pleural effusion must have positive cytology for M1/stage IV.

* It would be of value to know if the rupture of the capsule was spontaneous or caused by the surgeon, and if the source of malignant cells detected was peritoneal washings or ascites (FIGO note).

TNM: **T1a**
FIGO: IA

pT1a

Fig. 335

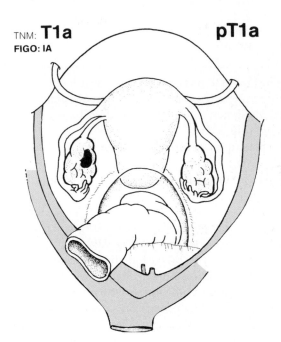

TNM: **T1b**
FIGO: IB

pT1b

Fig. 336

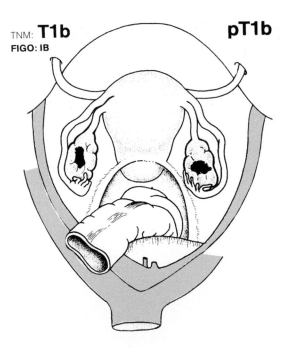

Fig. 337

TNM: **T1c**
FIGO: IC

TNM: **T1c**
FIGO: IC

T = pT

Ascites, peritoneal washing

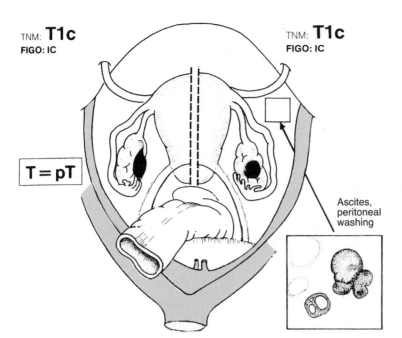

TNM: **T2a**
FIGO: IIA

pT2a

Fig. 338

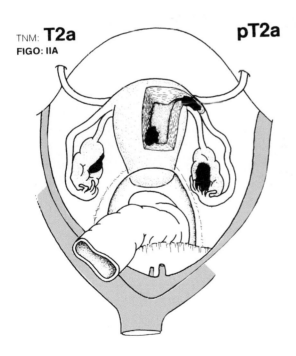

TNM: **T2b**
FIGO: IIB

pT2b

Fig. 339

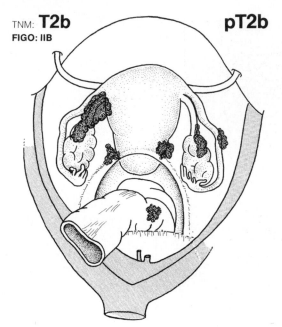

TNM: **T2c**
FIGO: IIC

pT2c

Fig. 340

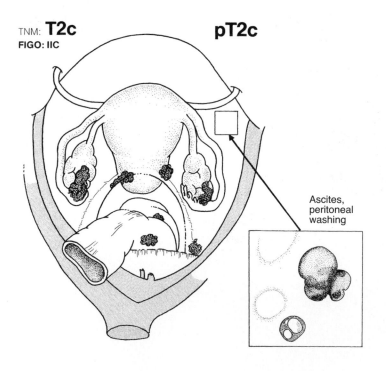

Ascites,
peritoneal
washing

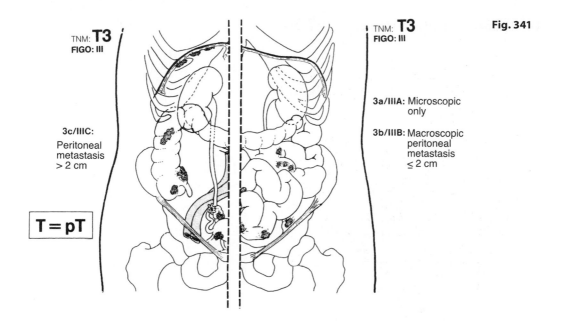

Fig. 341

TNM: **T3**
FIGO: III

TNM: **T3**
FIGO: III

3c/IIIC:
Peritoneal
metastasis
> 2 cm

3a/IIIA: Microscopic
only

3b/IIIB: Macroscopic
peritoneal
metastasis
≤ 2 cm

T = pT

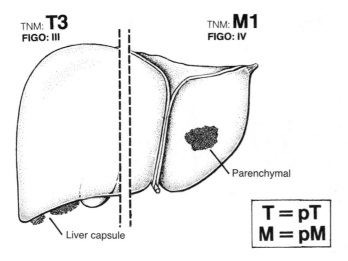

Fig. 342

TNM: **T3**
FIGO: III

TNM: **M1**
FIGO: IV

Parenchymal

Liver capsule

T = pT
M = pM

N – Regional Lymph Nodes

NX   Regional lymph nodes cannot be assessed
N0   No regional lymph node metastasis
N1   Regional lymph node metastasis (Fig. 343)

N1

pN1
FIGO: IIIC

Fig. 343

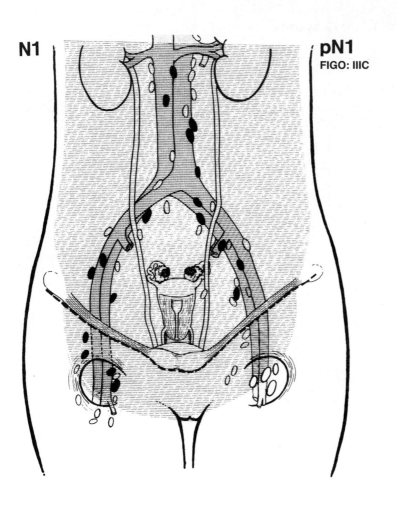

M – Distant Metastasis

MX   Distant metastasis cannot be assessed
M0   No distant metastasis
M1   Distant metastasis (Fig. 342, p. 261)

pTNM Pathological Classification

The pT, pN, and pM categories correspond to the T, N, and M categories.

pN0 Histological examination of a pelvic lymphadenectomy specimen will ordinarily include 10 or more lymph nodes. If the examined lymph nodes are negative, but the number ordinarily resected is not met, classify as pN0.

Fallopian Tube (ICD-O C57.0)

The definitions of the T, N, and M categories correspond to the FIGO stages. Both systems are included for comparison.

Rules for Classification

The classification applies only to carcinoma. There should be histological confirmation of the disease.

The FIGO stages are based on clinical staging. (TNM stages are based on clinical and/or pathological staging.)

Regional Lymph Nodes

The regional lymph nodes are the hypogastric (including obturator), common iliac, external iliac, lateral sacral, para-aortic, and inguinal nodes (see Fig. 334, p. 256)

TNM Clinical Classification

T – Primary Tumour

TNM categories	FIGO stages	
TX		Primary tumour cannot be assessed
T0		No evidence of primary tumour
Tis		Carcinoma in situ (preinvasive carcinoma)
T1	I	Tumour confined to fallopian tube(s)
T1a	IA	Tumour limited to one tube, without penetrating the serosal surface; no ascites (Fig. 344)

TNM categories	FIGO stages	
T1b	IB	Tumour limited to both tubes, without penetrating the serosal surface; no ascites (Fig. 345)
T1c	IC	Tumour limited to one or both tube(s) with extension onto or through the tubal serosa, or with malignant cells in ascites or peritoneal washings (Fig. 346)
T2	II	Tumour involves one or both fallopian tube(s) with pelvic extension
T2a	IIA	Extension and/or metastasis to uterus and/or ovaries (Fig. 347)
T2b	IIB	Extension to other pelvic structures (Fig. 348)
T2c	IIC	Pelvic extension (2a or 2b) with malignant cells in ascites or peritoneal washings (Fig. 349)
T3 and/ or N1	III	Tumour involves one or both fallopian tube(s) with peritoneal implants outside the pelvis and/or positive regional lymph nodes
T3a	IIIA	Microscopic peritoneal metastasis outside the pelvis (Figs. 341–343, pp 261–262)
T3b	IIIB	Macroscopic peritoneal metastasis outside the pelvis 2 cm or less in greatest dimension
T3c and/ or N1	IIIC	Peritoneal metastasis more than 2 cm in greatest dimension and/or positive regional lymph nodes (Fig. 343, p. 262)
M1	IV	Distant metastasis (excludes peritoneal metastasis) (Fig. 342, p. 261)

Note

Liver capsule metastasis is T3/stage III, liver parenchymal metastasis M1/stage IV. Pleural effusion must have positive cytology for M1/stage IV.

TNM: **T1a**
FIGO: IA

pT1a
FIGO: IA

Fig. 344

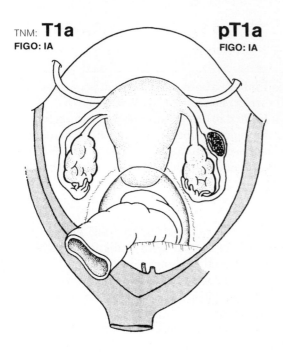

TNM: **T1b**
FIGO: IB

pT1b
FIGO: IB

Fig. 345

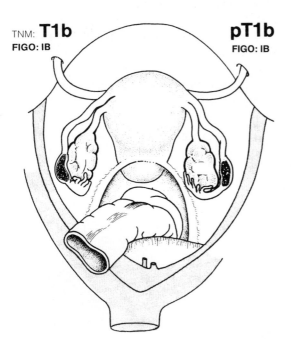

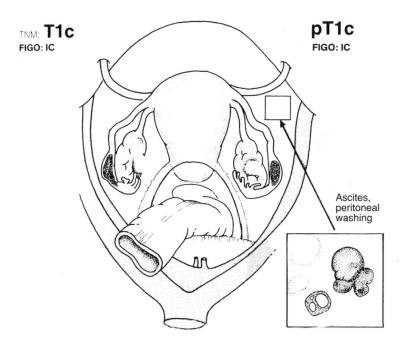

TNM: **T1c**
FIGO: IC

pT1c
FIGO: IC

Fig. 346

Ascites,
peritoneal
washing

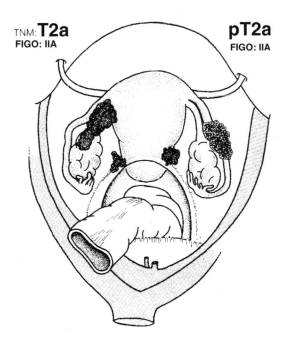

TNM: **T2a**
FIGO: IIA

pT2a
FIGO: IIA

Fig. 347

TNM: **T2b**
FIGO: IIB

pT2b
FIGO: IIB

Fig. 348

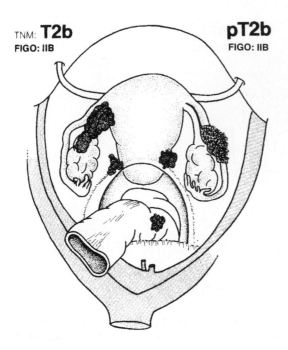

TNM: **T2c**
FIGO: IIC

pT2c
FIGO: IIC

Fig. 349

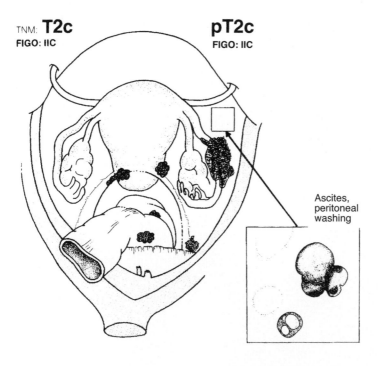

Ascites,
peritoneal
washing

N – Regional Lymph Nodes

NX   Regional lymph nodes cannot be assessed
N0   No regional lymph node metastasis
N1   Regional lymph node metastasis (Fig. 343, p. 262)

M – Distant Metastasis

MX   Distant metastasis cannot be assessed
M0   No distant metastasis
M1   Distant metastasis (Fig. 342, p. 261)

pTNM Pathological Classification

The pT, pN, and pM categories correspond to the T, N, and M categories.

pN0 Histological examination of a pelvic lymphadenectomy specimen will ordinarily include 10 or more lymph nodes. If the examined lymph nodes are negative, but the number ordinarily resected is not met, classify as pN0.

Gestational Trophoblastic Tumours

(ICD-O C58)

The following classification for gestational trophoblastic tumours is based on that of FIGO adopted in 1992 and updated in 2001 (Gestational trophoblastic tumours. Ngan HYS, Odicino F, Maisonneuve P, Beller U, Benedet JL, Heintz APM, Pecorelli S, Sideri M, Creasman WT. J Epidemiol Biostatist 2001; 6: 175–184).

The definitions of T and M categories correspond to the FIGO stages. Both systems are included for comparison. A prognostic scoring index, which is based on factors other than the anatomic extent of the disease, is used to assign cases to high risk and low risk categories, and these categories are used in stage grouping.

Rules for Classification

The classification applies to choriocarcinoma (9100/3), invasive hydatidiform mole (9100/1), and placental site trophoblastic tumour (9104/1). Placental site tumours should be reported separately. Histological confirmation is not required if the urine human chorionic gonadotropin (hCG) level is abnormally elevated. History of prior chemotherapy for this disease should be noted.

Editor's note:
This classification should also be applied to epitheloid trophoblastic tumour (ETT).

TM Clinical Classification

T–Primary Tumour/M–Distant Metastasis

TNM categories	FIGO stages	
TX		Primary tumour cannot be assessed
T0		No evidence of primary tumour
T1	I	Tumour confined to uterus (Fig. 350)
T2	II	Tumour extends to other genital structures: vagina, ovary, broad ligament, fallopian tube by metastasis or direct extension (Fig. 351)
M1a	III	Metastasis to lung(s)
M1b	IV	Other distant metastasis with or without lung involvement
		Note Stages I to IV are subdivided into A and B according to the prognostic score
Risk factors:		Age, antecedent pregnancy, months from index pregnancy, pretreatment serum hCG, largest tumour size including uterus, site of metastasis, number of metastasis, previous failed chemotherapy

Note
Genital metastasis (vagina, ovary, broad ligament, fallopran tube) is classified T2. Any involvement of non-genital structures, whether by direct invasion or metastasis is described using the M classification.

Gestational Trophoblastic Tumours (sidebar)

Prognostic score

Prognostic Faktor	0	1	2	4
Age	<40	≥40		
Antecedent Pregnancy	H. mole	Abortion	Term pregnancy	
Months from Index pregnancy	<4	4 – <7	7 – 12	>12
Pretreatment serum HCG (IU/ml)	$<10^3$	$10^3 – <10^4$	$10^4 – <10^5$	$\geq10^5$
Largest tumour size including uterus	<3 cm	3 – <5 cm	≥5 cm	
Sites of metastasis	Lung	Spleen, kidney	Gastro-intestinal tract	Liver, brain
Number of metastasis		1 – 4	5 – 8	>8
Previous failed therapy			Single drug	Two or more drugs

Risk categories:

Total prognostic score 7 or less = low risk (A)
Total score 8 or more = high risk (B)

Note
After publication of TNM 6th ed., FIGO changed their classification as follows. The FIGO stages will not be subdivided into A and B; instead, they recommend adding the total prognostic score to the stage (e.g., Stage III:4 instead of Stage IIIA); FIGO: ≤6 = low risk, ≥7 = high risk

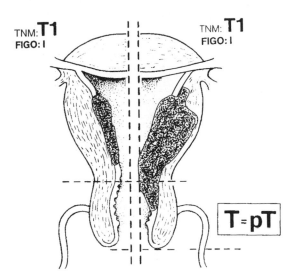

Fig. 350

TNM: **T1**
FIGO: I

TNM: **T1**
FIGO: I

T = pT

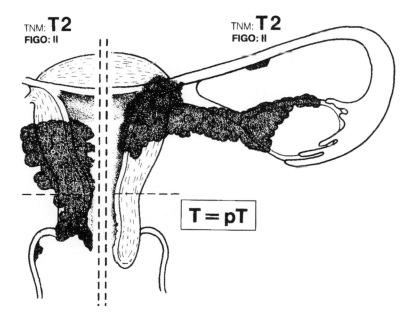

Fig. 351

TNM: **T2**
FIGO: II

TNM: **T2**
FIGO: II

T = pT

pTM Pathological Classification

The pT and pM categories correspond to the T and M categories.

Urological Tumours

Introductory Notes

The following sites are included:

- Penis
- Prostate
- Testis
- Kidney
- Renal pelvis and ureter
- Urinary bladder
- Urethra

Penis (ICD-O C60)

Rules for Classification

The classification applies only to carcinomas. There should be histological confirmation of the disease.

Anatomical Subsites (Fig. 352)

1. Prepuce (C60.0)
2. Glans penis (C60.1)
3. Body of penis (C60.2)

Regional Lymph Nodes

The regional lymph nodes are the superficial and deep inguinal and the pelvic nodes.

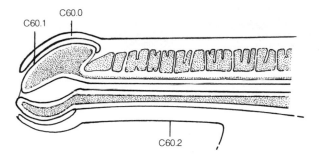

C60.1 C60.0

C60.2

Fig. 352

TN Clinical Classification

T – Primary Tumour

TX   Primary tumour cannot be assessed
T0   No evidence of primary tumour
Tis   Carcinoma in situ
Ta   Noninvasive verrucous carcinoma (Fig. 353)

T1   Tumour invades subepithelial connective tissue (Fig. 354)
T2   Tumour invades corpus spongiosum or cavernosum (Fig. 355)
T3   Tumour invades urethra (Fig. 356) or prostate (Fig. 357)
T4   Tumour invades other adjacent structures (Figs. 358, 359)

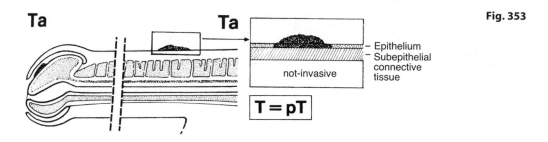

Fig. 353

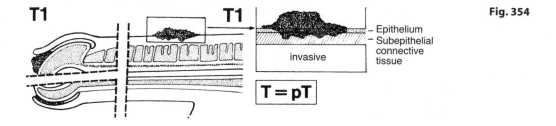

Fig. 354

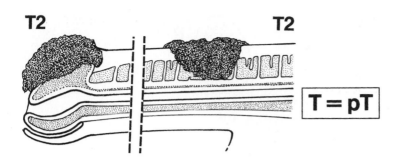

T2 **T2**

$$T = pT$$

Fig. 355

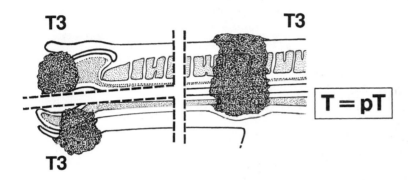

T3 **T3**

T3

$$T = pT$$

Fig. 356

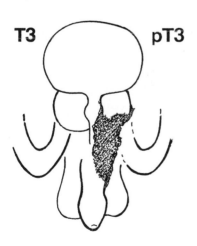

T3 **pT3**

Fig. 357

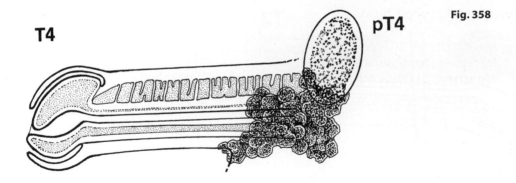

T4   **pT4**   **Fig. 358**

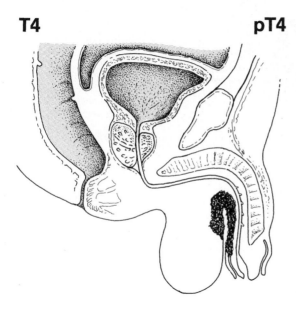

T4   **pT4**   **Fig. 359**

N – Regional Lymph Nodes

NX   Regional lymph nodes cannot be assessed
N0   No regional lymph node metastasis
N1   Metastasis in a single superficial inguinal lymph node (Fig. 360)

N1   **pN1**   **Fig. 360**

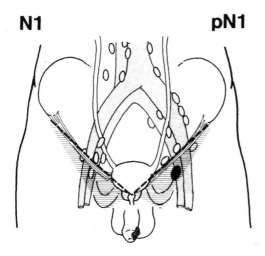

N2   Metastasis in multiple (Fig. 361) or bilateral superficial inguinal lymph nodes (Fig. 362)

N2   **pN2**   Fig. 361

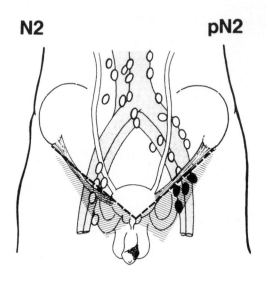

N2   **pN2**   Fig. 362

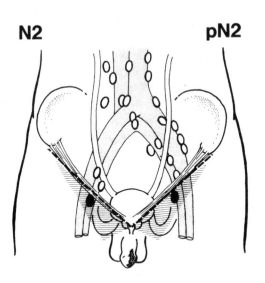

N3   Metastasis in deep inguinal (Fig. 363) or pelvic lymph node(s), unilateral (Fig. 364) or
      bilateral (Fig. 365)

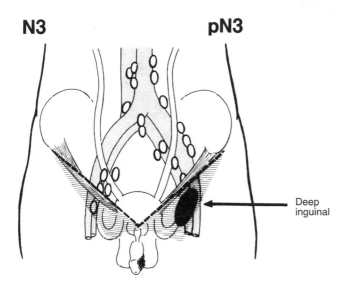

N3   **pN3**   **Fig. 363**

Deep
inguinal

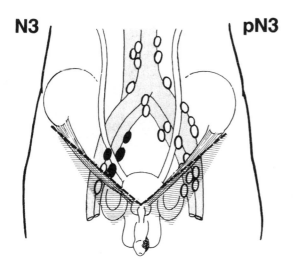

N3   **pN3**   **Fig. 364**

N3 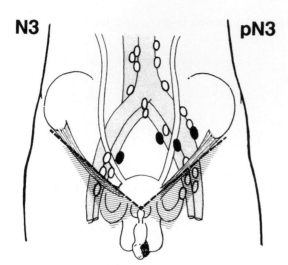 pN3

Fig. 365

pTN Pathological Classification

The pT and pN categories correspond to the T and N categories.

Prostate (ICD-O C61) (Figs. 366, 418, p. 321)

Rules for Classification

The classification applies only to adenocarcinomas. Transitional cell carcinoma of the prostate is classified as a urethral tumour (see p. 327 ff.). There should be histological confirmation of the disease.

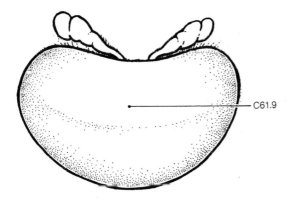

Fig. 366

C61.9

Regional Lymph Nodes (Fig. 367)

The regional lymph nodes are the nodes of the true pelvis, which essentially are the pelvic nodes below the bifurcation of the common iliac arteries. Laterality does not affect the N classification.

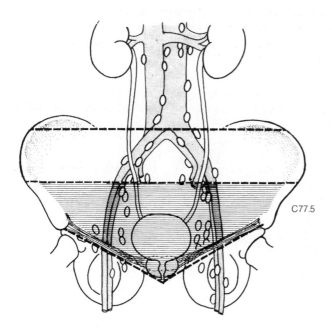

Fig. 367

C77.5

TN Clinical Classification

T – Primary Tumour

TX   Primary tumour cannot be assessed

T0   No evidence of primary tumour

T1   Clinically inapparent tumour not palpable or visible by imaging (Fig. 368)

    T1a   Tumour incidental histological finding in 5% or less of tissue resected

    T1b   Tumour incidental histological finding in more than 5% of tissue resected

    T1c   Tumour identified by needle biopsy (e.g. because of elevated PSA)

T2   Tumour confined within the prostate[1]

    T2a   Tumour involves one half of one lobe or less (Fig. 369)

    T2b   Tumour involves more than one half of one lobe, but not both lobes (Fig. 369)

    T2c   Tumour involves both lobes (Fig. 370)

Notes

[1] Tumour found in one or both lobes by needle biopsy, but not palpable or visible by imaging, is classified as T1c.

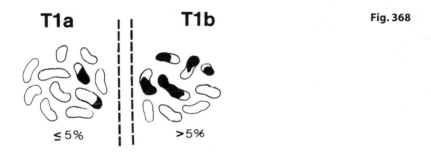

T1a   **T1b**

≤ 5%   >5%

Fig. 368

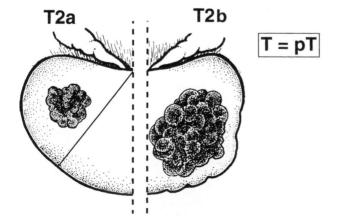

T2a   **T2b**

T = pT

Fig. 369

T3   Tumour extends through the prostatic capsule[2]
    T3a   Extracapsular extension (unilateral or bilateral) (Figs. 371, 372)
    T3b   Tumour invades seminal vesicle(s) (Fig. 373)

Note
[2] Invasion into the prostatic apex or into (but not beyond) the prostatic capsule is not classified as T3, but as T2.

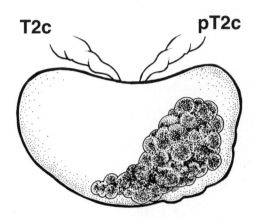

Fig. 370

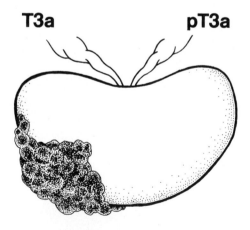

Fig. 371

T3a   pT3a   Fig. 372

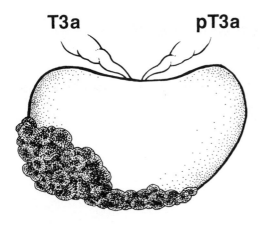

T3b   pT3b   Fig. 373

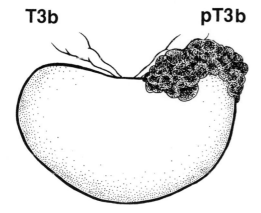

T4   Tumour is fixed or invades adjacent structures other than seminal vesicles: bladder neck, external sphincter, rectum, levator muscles, and/or pelvic wall (Figs. 374, 375)

T4   **pT4**   **Fig. 374**

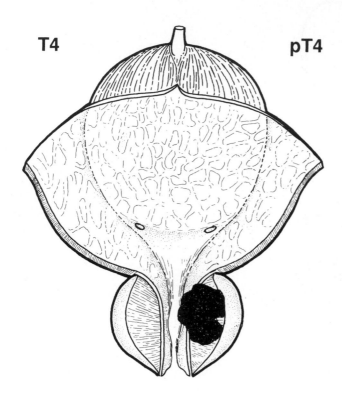

T4 **pT4** Fig. 375

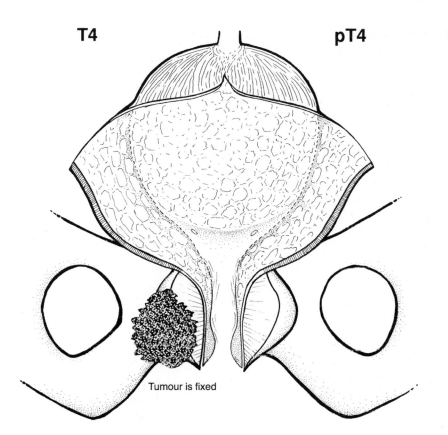

Tumour is fixed

N – Regional Lymph Nodes

NX   Regional lymph nodes cannot be assessed
N0   No regional lymph node metastasis
N1   Regional lymph node metastasis (Fig. 376, 377)

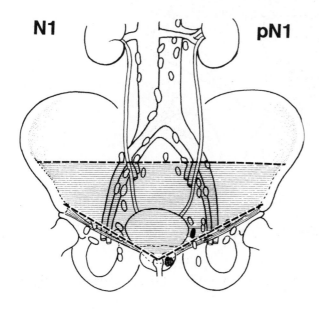

N1   pN1   Fig. 376

N1 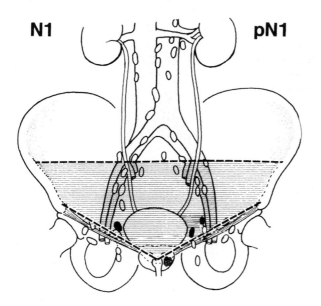 pN1

Fig. 377

pTN: Pathological Classification

The pT and pN categories correspond to the T and N categories.

However, there is no pT1 category because there is insufficient tissue to assess the highest pT category.

Note

Metastasis no larger than 0.2 cm can be designated pN1(mi).

Testis (ICD-O C62) (Fig. 378)

Rules for Classification

The classification applies only to germ cell tumours of the testis. There should be histological confirmation of the disease and division of cases by histological type.

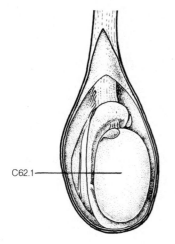

Fig. 378

C62.1

Regional Lymph Nodes (Fig. 379)

The regional lymph nodes are the abdominal para-aortic (periaortic), preaortic, interaorto-caval, precaval, paracaval, retrocaval, and retroaortic nodes. Nodes along the spermatic vein should be considered regional. Laterality does not affect the N classification. The intrapelvic nodes and the inguinal nodes are considered regional after scrotal or inguinal surgery.

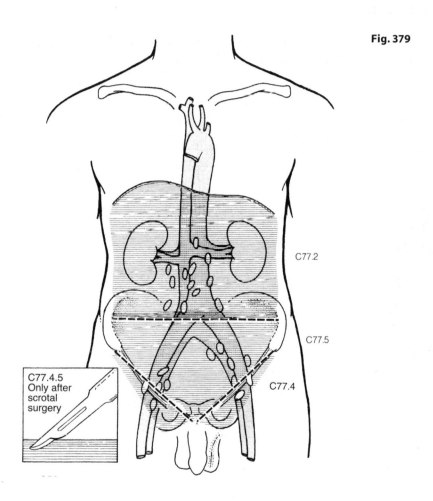

Fig. 379

C77.2

C77.5

C77.4

C77.4.5
Only after
scrotal
surgery

TN Clinical Classification

T – Primary tumour

Except for pTis and pT4, where radical orchiectomy is not always necessary for classification purposes, the extent of the primary tumour is classified after radical orchiectomy; see pT. In other circumstances, TX is used if no radical orchiectomy has been performed.

N – Regional Lymph Nodes

NX   Regional lymph nodes cannot be assessed
N0   No regional lymph node metastasis
N1   Metastasis with a lymph node mass 2 cm or less in greatest dimension or multiple lymph nodes, none more than 2 cm in greatest dimension (Figs. 380 – 385)
N2   Metastasis with a lymph node mass more than 2 cm but not more than 5 cm in greatest dimension, or multiple lymph nodes, any one mass more than 2 cm but not more than 5 cm in greatest dimension (Figs. 386 – 388)
N3   Metastasis with a lymph node mass more than 5 cm in greatest dimension (Figs. 389 – 392)

N1   **pN1**   Fig. 380

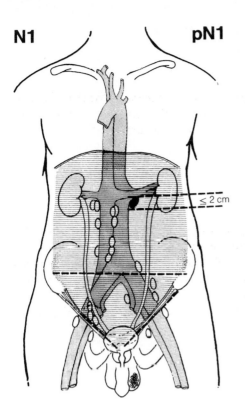

≤ 2 cm

N1   **pN1**   Fig. 381

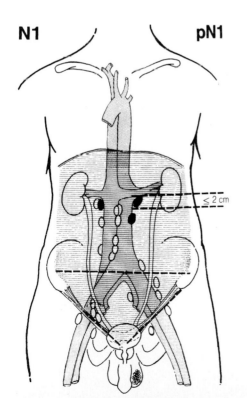

≤ 2 cm

Testis

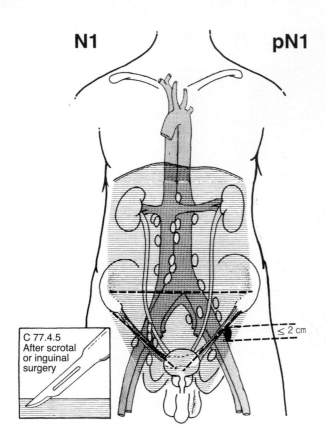

N1

pN1

Fig. 382

C 77.4.5
After scrotal
or inguinal
surgery

≤ 2 cm

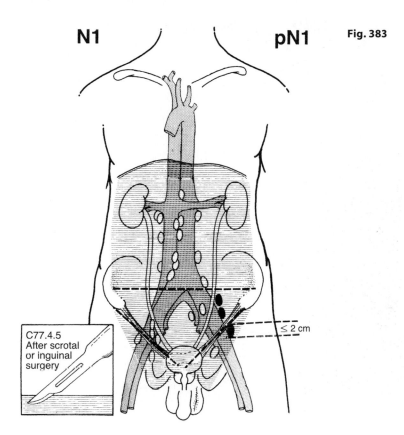

N1   **pN1**   Fig. 383

C77.4.5
After scrotal
or inguinal
surgery

≤ 2 cm

Testis

N1   **pN2**   Fig. 384

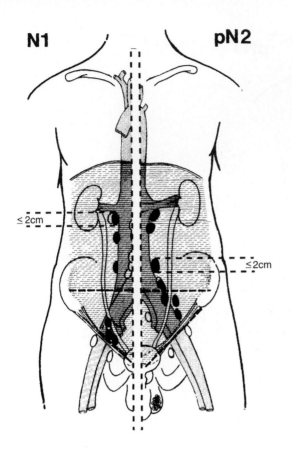

≤ 2cm

≤2cm

N1

pN2

Fig. 385

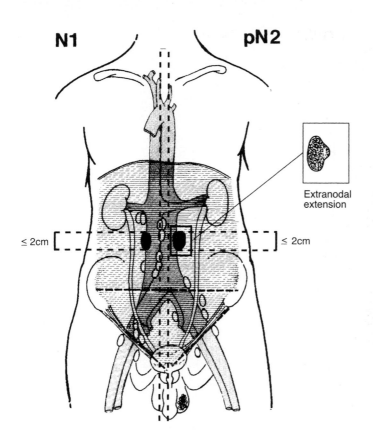

Extranodal
extension

≤ 2cm

≤ 2cm

Testis

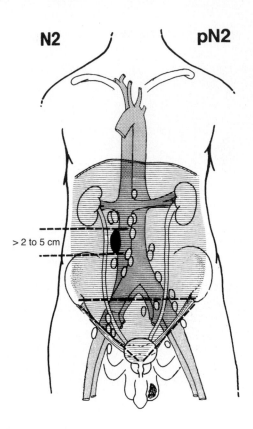

N2   **pN2**   Fig. 386

> 2 to 5 cm

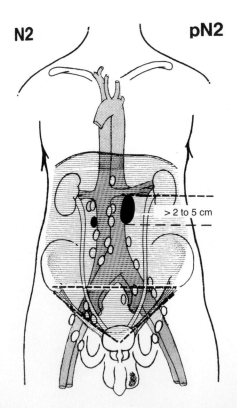

N2   **pN2**   Fig. 387

> 2 to 5 cm

N2

pN2

Fig. 388

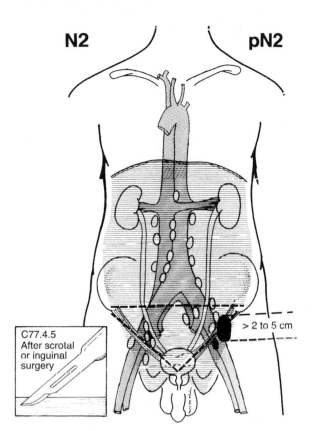

C77.4.5
After scrotal
or inguinal
surgery

> 2 to 5 cm

Testis

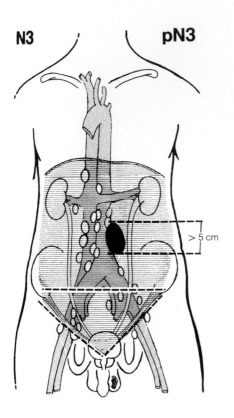

N3   pN3   **Fig. 389**

> 5 cm

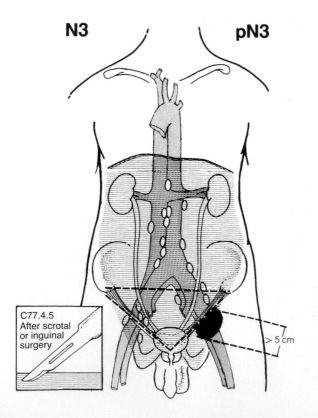

N3   pN3   **Fig. 390**

C77.4.5
After scrotal
or inguinal
surgery

> 5 cm

N3   **pN3**

Fig. 391

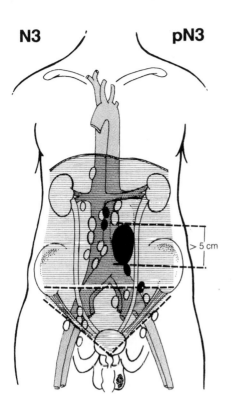

> 5 cm

N3   **pN3**

Fig. 392

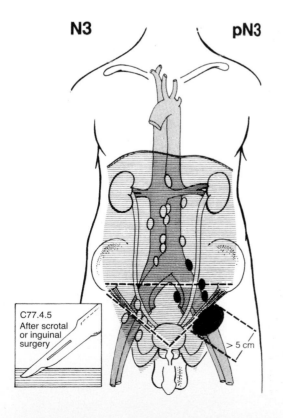

C77.4.5
After scrotal
or inguinal
surgery

> 5 cm

pTN Pathological Classification

pT – Primary Tumour

pTX   Primary tumour cannot be assessed (if no radical orchiectomy is performed TX is used))
pT0   No evidence of primary tumour (e.g., histologic scar in testis)
pTis   Intratubular germ cell neoplasia (carcinoma in situ)

pT1   Tumour limited to testis and epididymis without vascular/lymphatic invasion; tumour may invade tunica albuginea but not tunica vaginalis (Fig. 393)
pT2   Tumour limited to testis and epididymis with vascular/lymphatic invasion (Fig. 393), or tumour extending through tunica albuginea with involvement of tunica vaginalis (Fig. 394)

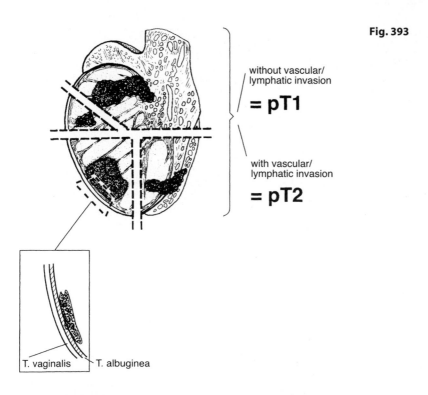

Fig. 393

without vascular/
lymphatic invasion

= pT1

with vascular/
lymphatic invasion

= pT2

T. vaginalis   T. albuginea

pT2

Fig. 394

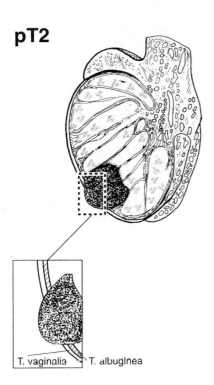

T. vaginalis   T. albuginea

pT3   Tumour invades spermatic cord with or without vascular/lymphatic invasion (Fig. 395)

pT4   Tumour invades scrotum with or without vascular/lymphatic invasion (Fig. 396)

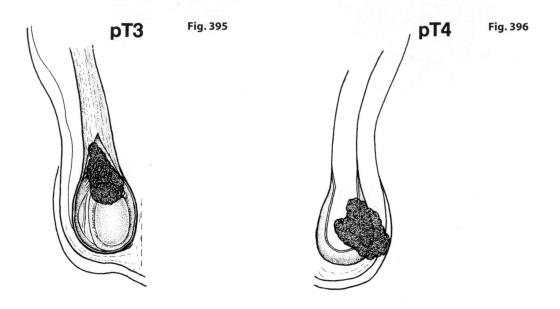

pT3   Fig. 395

pT4   Fig. 396

pN – Regional Lymph Nodes

pNX   Regional lymph nodes cannot be assessed

pN0   No regional lymph node metastasis

pN1   Metastasis with a lymph node mass 2 cm or less in greatest dimension and 5 or fewer positive nodes, none more than 2 cm in greatest dimension (Fig. 380–383, pp. 295–297)

pN2   Metastasis with a lymph node mass (Fig. 384–388, pp. 298–301) more than 2 cm but not more than 5 cm in greatest dimension; or more than 5 nodes positive, none more than 5 cm; or evidence of extranodal extension of tumour (Fig. 385, p. 299)

pN3   Metastasis with a lymph node mass more than 5 cm in greatest dimension (Fig. 389–392, pp. 302–303)

Kidney (ICD-O C64) (Fig. 397)

Rules for Classification

The classification applies only to renal cell carcinoma. There should be histological confirmation of the disease.

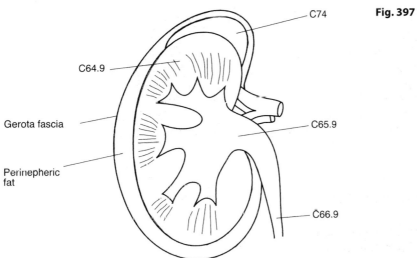

Fig. 397

Regional Lymph Nodes (Fig. 398)

The regional lymph nodes are the hilar, abdominal para-aortic (periaortic), preaortic, inter-aortocaval, precaval, paracaval, retrocaval and retroaortic nodes. Laterality does not affect the N categories.

Fig. 398

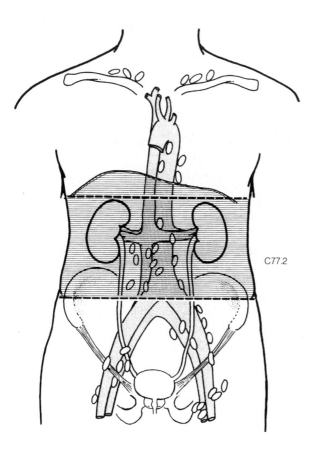

C77.2

TN Clinical Classification

T – Primary Tumour

TX   Primary tumour cannot be assessed
T0   No evidence of primary tumour

T1   Tumour 7.0 cm or less in greatest dimension, limited to the kidney
        T1a   Tumour 4.0 cm or less in greatest dimensinon (Fig. 399)
        T1b   Tumour more than 4.0 cm but not more than 7.0 cm in greatest dimension
             (Fig. 400)

T1a   pT1a   Fig. 399

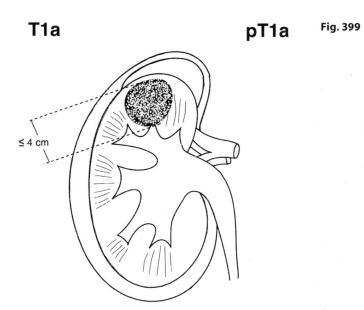

≤ 4 cm

T1b   **pT1b**   Fig. 400

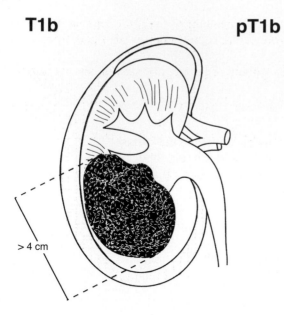

> 4 cm

T2   Tumour more than 7.0 cm in greatest dimension, limited to the kidney (Fig. 401)

T3   Tumour extends into major veins or directly invades adrenal gland or perinephric tissues but not beyond Gerota fascia

     T3a   Tumour directly invades adrenal gland or perinephric tissues[1] but not beyond Gerota fascia (Fig. 402)

     T3b   Tumour grossly extends into renal vein(s)[2] or vena cava below diaphragm (Fig. 403)

     T3c   Tumour grossly extends into vena cava above diaphragm (Fig. 404)

Notes

[1] Includes renal sinus (peripelvic) fat

[2] Includes segmental (muscle-containing) branches

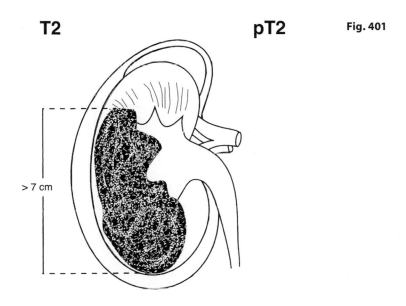

T2   **pT2**   **Fig. 401**

> 7 cm

Kidney

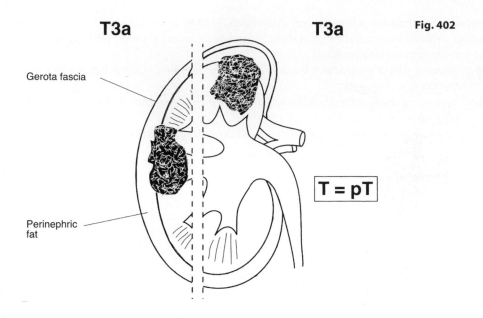

T3a   **T3a**   Fig. 402

Gerota fascia

Perinephric fat

$T = pT$

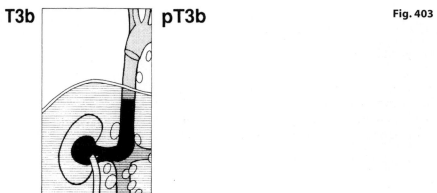

T3b   **pT3b**   Fig. 403

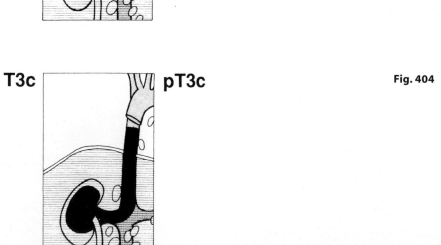

T3c   **pT3c**   Fig. 404

T4   Tumour directly invades beyond Gerota fascia (Fig. 405)

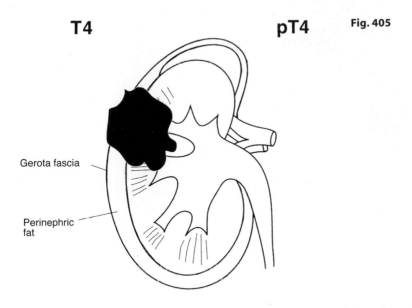

T4   **pT4**   **Fig. 405**

Gerota fascia

Perinephric
fat

N – Regional Lymph Nodes

NX   Regional lymph nodes cannot be assessed
N0   No regional lymph node metastasis
N1   Metastasis in a single regional lymph node (Fig. 406)
N2   Metastasis in more than one regional lymph node (Fig. 407)

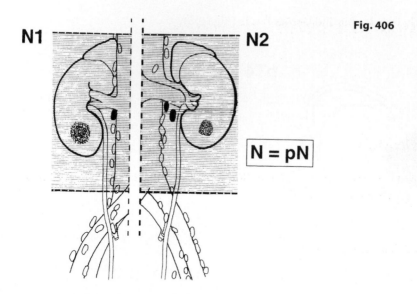

Fig. 406

$N = pN$

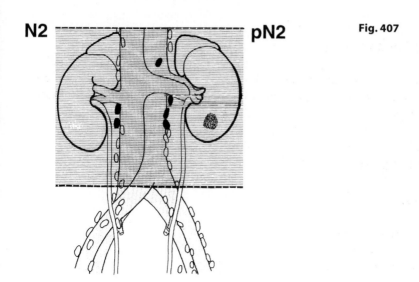

Fig. 407

pTN Pathological Classification

The pT and pN categories correspond to the T and N categories.

Kidney

Renal Pelvis and Ureter (ICD-O C65, C66)

Rules for Classification

The classification applies only to carcinomas. Papilloma is excluded. There should be histological or cytological confirmation of the disease.

Anatomical Sites (Fig. 397, p. 307)

1. Renal pelvis (C65.9)
2. Ureter (C66.9)

Regional Lymph Nodes (Fig. 399, p. 308)

The regional lymph nodes are the hilar, abdominal para-aortic (periaortic), preaortic, interaortocaval, retrocaval amd retroaortic nodes, and, for ureter, intrapelvic nodes. Laterality does not affect the N classification.

TN Clinical Classification

T – Primary Tumour

TX   Primary tumour cannot be assessed
T0   No evidence of primary tumour
Ta   Noninvasive papillary carcinoma (Fig. 408)
Tis   Carcinoma in situ

T1   Tumour invades subepithelial connective tissue (Fig. 408)
T2   Tumour invades muscularis (Fig. 408)
T3   *(Renal pelvis)* Tumour invades beyond muscularis into peripelvic fat or renal parenchyma (Fig. 409)
        (Ureter) Tumour invades beyond muscularis into periureteric fat (Fig. 409)

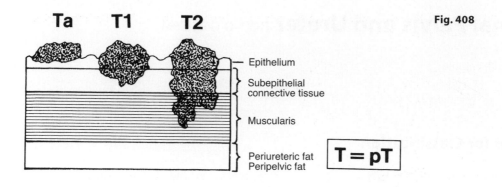

Fig. 408

Ta   T1   T2

Epithelium

Subepithelial
connective tissue

Muscularis

Periureteric fat
Peripelvic fat

T = pT

Fig. 409

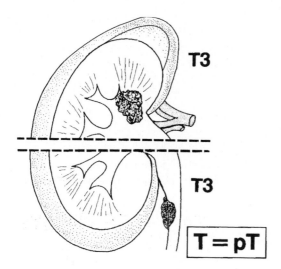

T3

T3

T = pT

T4   Tumour invades adjacent organs (Figs. 410, 411) or through the kidney into perine-
       phric fat (Fig. 412)

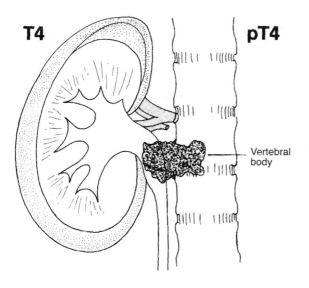

Fig. 410

Vertebral
body

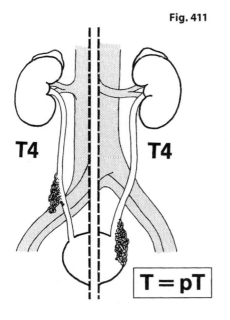

Fig. 411

T = pT

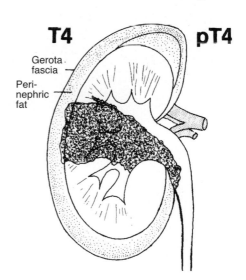

Fig. 412

Gerota
fascia

Peri-
nephric
fat

N – Regional Lymph Nodes

NX   Regional lymph nodes cannot be assessed
N0   No regional lymph node metastasis
N1   Metastasis in a single lymph node 2 cm or less in greatest dimension (Fig. 413)
N2   Metastasis in a single lymph node more than 2 cm but not more than 5 cm in greatest dimension (Fig. 414), or multiple lymph nodes, none more than 5 cm in greatest dimension (Fig. 415)
N3   Metastasis in a lymph node more than 5 cm in greatest dimension (Figs. 416, 417)

N1   **pN1**   Fig. 413

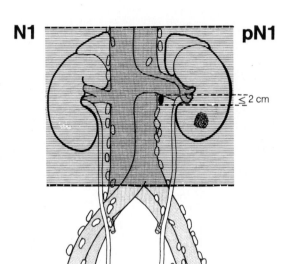

≦ 2 cm

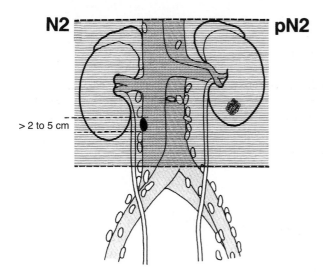

N2   pN2

> 2 to 5 cm

Fig. 414

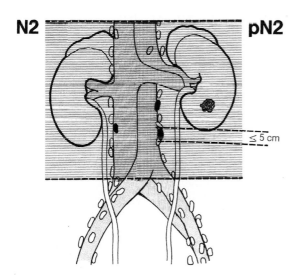

N2   pN2

≤ 5 cm

Fig. 415

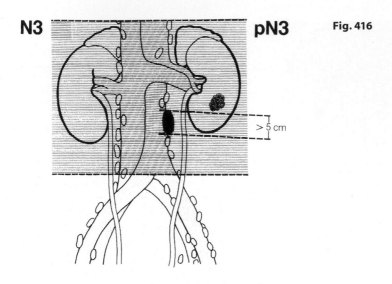

Fig. 416

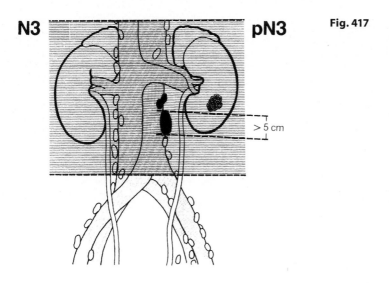

Fig. 417

pTN Pathological Classification

The pT and pN categories correspond to the T and N categories.

Urinary Bladder (ICD-O C67)

Rules for Classification

The classification applies only to carcinomas. Papilloma is excluded. There should be histological or cytological confirmation of the disease.

Anatomical Subsites (Fig. 418)

1. Trigone (C67.0)
2. Dome (C67.1)
3. Lateral wall (C67.2)
4. Anterior wall (C67.3)
5. Posterior wall (C67.4)
6. Bladder neck (C67.5)
7. Ureteric orifice (C67.6)
8. Urachus (C67.7)

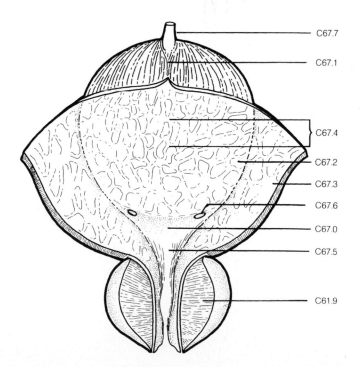

Fig. 418

C67.7
C67.1
C67.4
C67.2
C67.3
C67.6
C67.0
C67.5
C61.9

Urinary Bladder

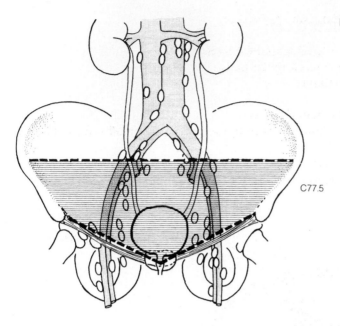

Fig. 419

C77.5

Regional Lymph Nodes (Fig. 419)

The regional lymph nodes are the nodes of the true pelvis, which essentially are the pelvic nodes below the bifurcation of the common iliac arteries. Laterality does not affect the N classification.

TN Clinical Classification

T – Primary Tumour (Fig. 420)

The suffix (m) should be added to the appropriate T category to indicate multiple tumours. The suffix (is) may be added to any T to indicate presence of associated carcinoma in situ.

TX   Primary tumour cannot be assessed
T0   No evidence of primary tumour
Ta   Noninvasive papillary carcinoma
Tis   Carcinoma in situ: "flat tumour"

T1   Tumour invades subepithelial connective tissue
T2   Tumour invades muscle
      T2a   Tumour invades superficial muscle (inner half)
      T2b   Tumour invades deep muscle (outer half)
T3   Tumour invades perivesical tissue:
      T3a   Microscopically
      T3b   Macroscopically (extravesical mass)
T4   Tumour invades any of the following: prostate, uterus, vagina, pelvic wall, abdominal wall
      T4a   Tumour invades prostate or uterus or vagina
      T4b   Tumour invades pelvic wall or abdominal wall

1 - Epithelium
2 - Subepithelial connective tissue
3 - Muscle
4 - Perivesical fat

Fig. 420

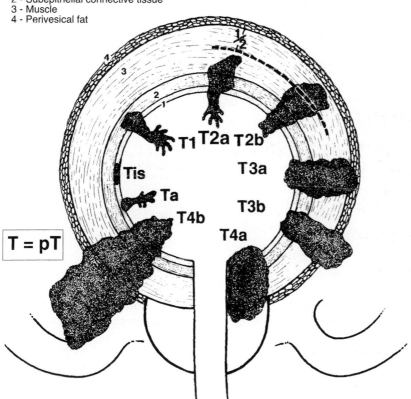

N – Regional Lymph Nodes

NX   Regional lymph nodes cannot be assessed
N0   No regional lymph node metastasis
N1   Metastasis in a single lymph node 2 cm or less in greatest dimension (Fig. 421)
N2   Metastasis in a single lymph node more than 2 cm but not more than 5 cm in greatest dimension (Fig. 422), or multiple lymph nodes, none more than 5 cm in greatest dimension (Fig. 423)
N3   Metastasis in a lymph node more than 5 cm in greatest dimension (Figs. 424, 425)

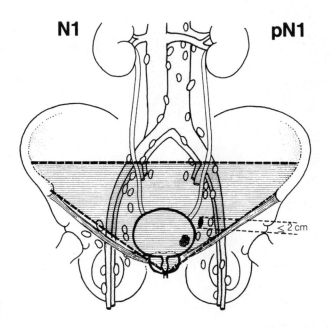

N1   pN1   Fig. 421

≤ 2 cm

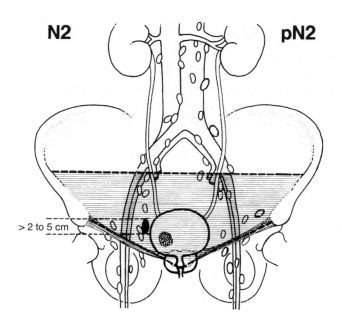

N2

pN2

Fig. 422

> 2 to 5 cm

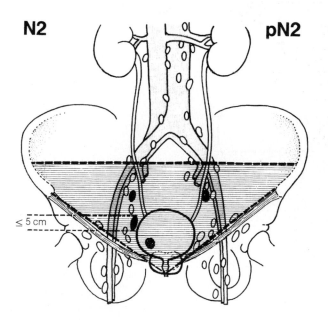

N2

pN2

Fig. 423

≤ 5 cm

N3   **pN3**   Fig. 424

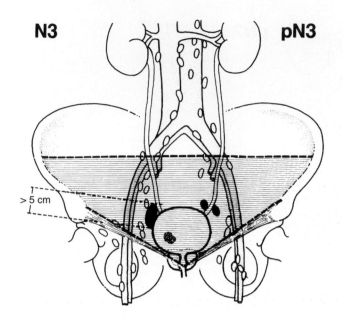

> 5 cm

N3   **pN3**   Fig. 425

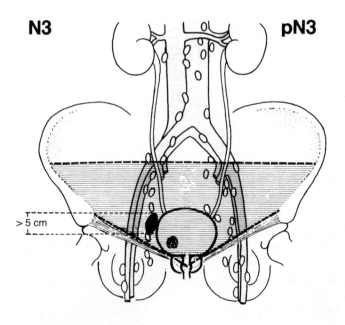

> 5 cm

pTN Pathological Classification

The pT and pN categories correspond to the T and N categories.

Urethra

Rules for Classification

The classification applies to carcinomas of the urethra (ICD-O C68.0) and transitional cell carcinomas of the prostate (ICD-O C61.9) and prostatic urethra. There should be histological or cytological confirmation of the disease.

Regional Lymph Nodes (Fig. 419, p. 322)

The regional lymph nodes are the inguinal and the pelvic nodes. Laterality does not affect the N classification.

TN Clinical Classification

T – Primary Tumour

TX   Primary tumour cannot be assessed
T0   No evidence of primary tumour

Urethra (male and female)

Ta   Noninvasive papillary, polypoid, or verrucous carcinoma (Figs. 426, 427)
Tis   Carcinoma in situ

T1   Tumour invades subepithelial connective tissue (Figs. 426, 428)
T2   Tumour invades any of the following: corpus spongiosum, prostate, periurethral muscle (Figs. 426, 429, 430)
T3   Tumour invades any of the following: corpus cavernosum, beyond prostatic capsule, anterior vagina, bladder neck (Figs. 431–433)
T4   Tumour invades other adjacent organs (Fig. 434)

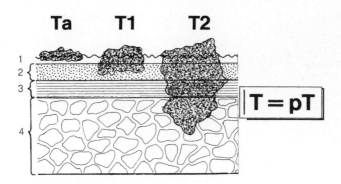

Fig. 426. *1* Epithelium, *2* subepithelial connective tissue, *3* urethral muscle, *4* urogenital diaphragm

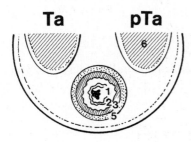

Fig. 427. *1* Epithelium, *2* subepithelial connective tissue, *3* urethral muscle, *5* corpus spongiosum, *6* corpus cavernosum

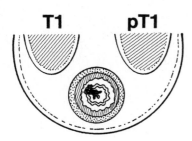

Fig. 428

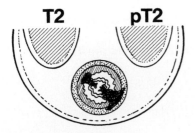

Fig. 429

Urethra

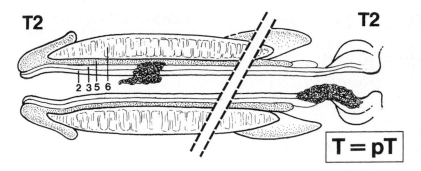

Fig. 430. *2,3,5,6:*
See Fig. 427

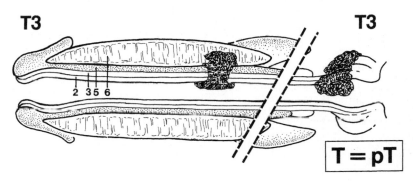

Fig. 431. *2,3,5,6:*
See Fig. 427

T3   **pT3**   Fig. 432

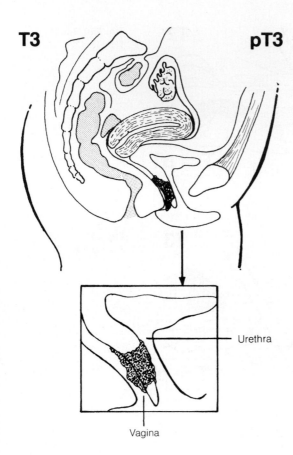

Urethra

Vagina

T3

pT3

Fig. 433

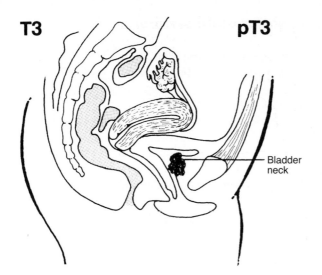

Bladder
neck

T4

pT4

Fig. 434

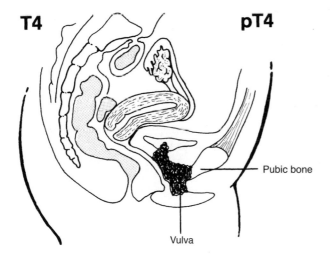

Pubic bone

Vulva

Transitional cell carcinoma of prostate (prostatic urethra)

Tis pu   Carcinoma in situ, involvement of prostatic urethra (Fig. 435)
Tis pd   Carcinoma in situ, involvement of prostatic ducts (Fig. 436)

T1   Tumour invades subepithelial connective tissue (Figs. 435, 436)
T2   Tumour invades any of the following: prostatic stroma, corpus spongiosum, periure-
      thral muscle (Figs. 436, 437)
T3   Tumour invades any of the following: corpus cavernosum, beyond prostatic capsule,
      bladder neck (extraprostatic extension) (Fig. 438)
T4   Tumour invades other adjacent organs (invasion of the bladder) (Fig. 439)

Fig. 435

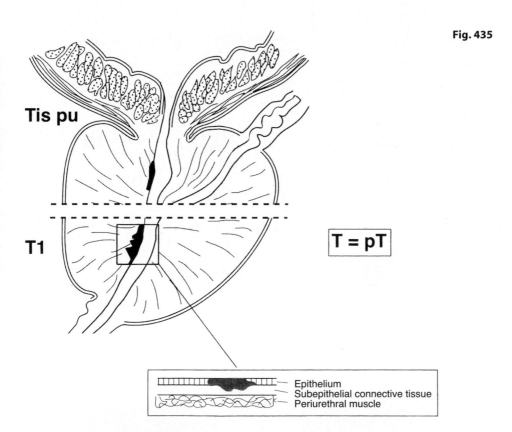

Tis pu

T1

T = pT

Epithelium
Subepithelial connective tissue
Periurethral muscle

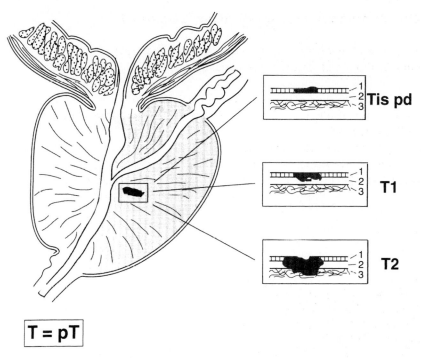

Fig. 436. *1* Epithelium, *2* subepithelial connective tissue, *3* prostatic stroma

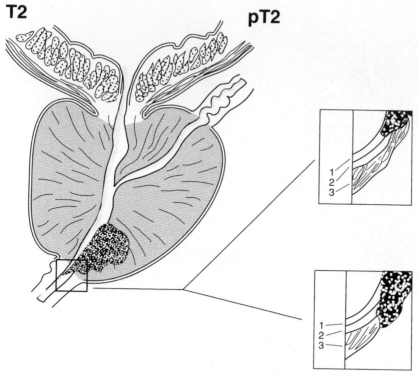

Fig. 437. *1* Urethral epithelium and subepithelial connective tissue, *2* periurethral muscle, *3* corpus spongiosum

Fig. 438

T3

pT3

Bladder neck

Beyond prostatic capsule
Corpus cavernosum

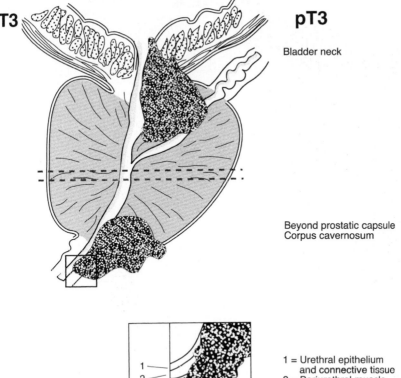

1 = Urethral epithelium
    and connective tissue
2 = Periurethral muscle
3 = Corpus spongiosum
4 = Corpus cavernosum

T4

pT4   **Fig. 439**

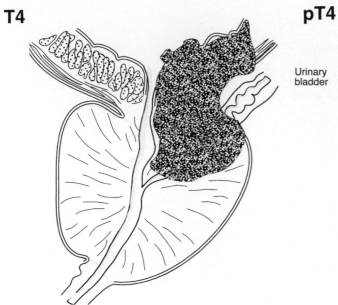

Urinary
bladder

N – Regional Lymph Nodes

NX Regional lymph nodes cannot be assessed
N0 No regional lymph node metastasis
N1 Metastasis in a single lymph node 2 cm or less in greatest dimension (Fig. 440)

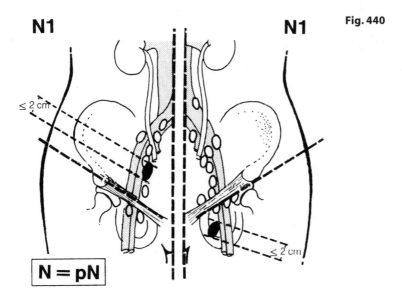

Fig. 440

N2   Metastasis in a single lymph node more than 2 cm in greatest dimension (Fig. 441), or multiple lymph nodes (Fig. 442)

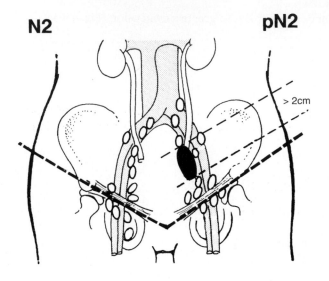

N2   **pN2**   **Fig. 441**

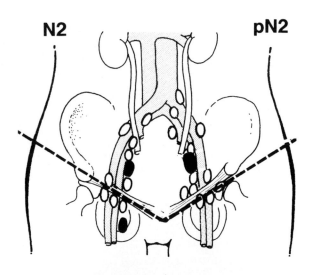

N2   **pN2**   **Fig. 442**

pTN Pathological Classification

The pT and pN categories correspond to the T and N categories.

Ophthalmic Tumours

Introductory Notes

Tumours of the eye and its adnexa are a disparate group including carcinoma, melanoma, sarcomas, and retinoblastoma. For clinical convenience they are classified in one section.

Tumours in the following sites are classified:

- Eyelid (eyelid melanoma is classified with skin tumours)
- Conjunctiva
- Uvea
- Retina
- Orbit
- Lacrimal gland

Regional Lymph Nodes (Fig. 443)

The regional lymph nodes are the preauricular (1), submandibular (2) and cervical (3) lymph nodes.

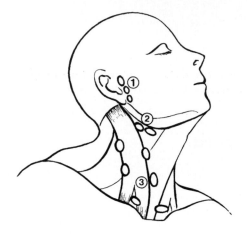

Fig. 443

The definitions of N and M categories for ophthalmic tumours are:

N – Regional Lymph Nodes

NX   Regional lymph nodes cannot be assessed
N0   No regional lymph node metastasis
N1   Regional lymph node metastasis

Carcinoma of Eyelid (ICD-O C44.1)

Rules of Classification

There should be histological confirmation of the disease and division of cases by histological type, e.g., basal cell, squamous cell, sebaceous carcinoma.

T Clinical Classification

T – Primary Tumour

TX   Primary tumour cannot be assessed
T0   No evidence of primary tumour
Tis   Carcinoma in situ

T1   Tumour of any size, not invading the tarsal plate; or at eyelid margin, 5.0 mm or less in greatest dimension (Fig. 444a,b)

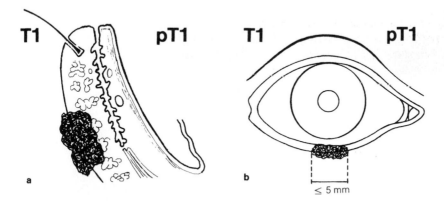

Fig. 444a, b

T2   Tumour invades tarsal plate; or at eyelid margin, more than 5.0 mm but not more than 10.0 mm in greatest dimension (Fig. 445a,b)

T3   Tumour involves full eyelid thickness; or at eyelid margin, more than 10.0 mm in greatest dimension (Fig. 446a,b)

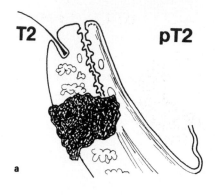

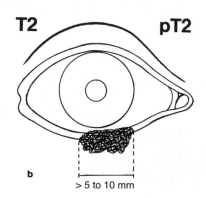

Fig. 445a, b

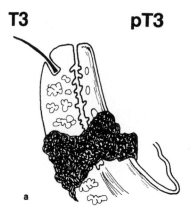

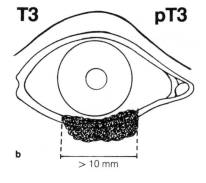

Fig. 446a, b

T4   Tumour invades adjacent structures, which include bulbar conjunctiva, sclera/globe, soft tissues of the orbit, perineural invasion, bone/periosteum of the orbit, nasal cavity/paranasal sinuses, and central nervous system (Fig. 447a,b)

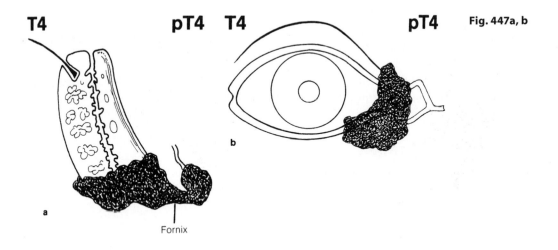

Fig. 447a, b

Fornix

pT Pathological Classification

The pT categories correspond to the T categories.

Carcinoma of Conjunctiva (ICD-O C 69.0)

Rules for Classification

There should be histological confirmation of the disease and division of cases by histological type, e.g., mucoepidermoid and squamous cell carcinoma.

T Clinical Classification

T – Primary Tumour

TX   Primary tumour cannot be assessed
T0   No evidence of primary tumour
Tis   Carcinoma in situ

T1   Tumour 5.0 mm or less in greatest dimension (Fig. 448)
T2   Tumour more than 5.0 mm in greatest dimension, without invasion of adjacent structures (Fig. 449)

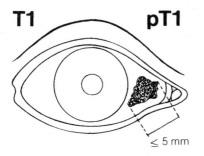

Fig. 448

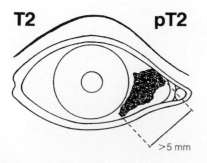

Fig. 449

T3   Tumour invades adjacent structures, excluding the orbit (Fig. 450)
T4   Tumour invades the orbit
     T4a   Tumour invades orbital soft tissues, without bone invasion (Fig. 451a,b)

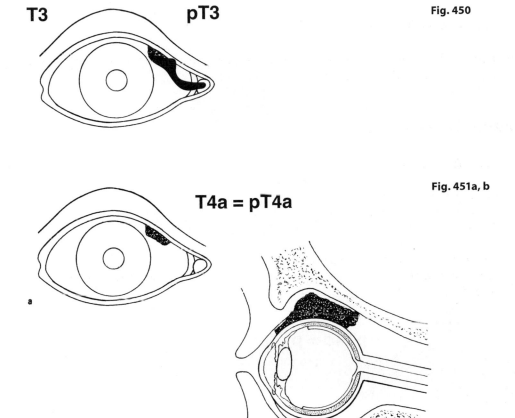

T3   **pT3**

Fig. 450

T4a = pT4a

Fig. 451a, b

a

b

T4b   Tumour invades bone (Fig. 452a,b)
T4c   Tumour invades paranasal sinuses (Fig. 453a,b)

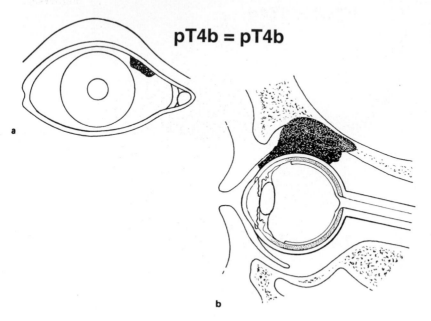

pT4b = pT4b

Fig. 452a, b

a

b

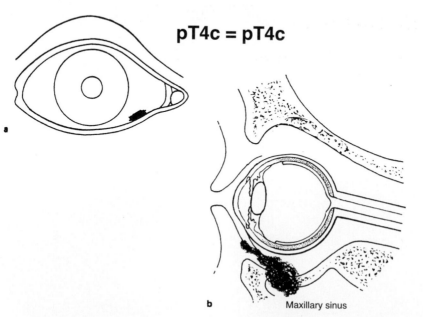

pT4c = pT4c

Fig. 453a, b

a

b   Maxillary sinus

T4d   Tumour invades brain (Fig. 454a,b)

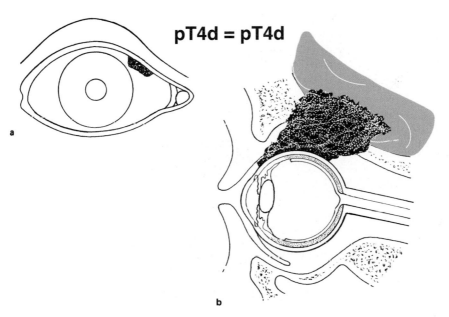

pT4d = pT4d

a

b

pT Pathological Classification

The pT categories correspond to the T categories.

Malignant Melanoma of Conjunctiva (ICD-O C69.0)

Rules for Classification

The classification applies only to malignant melanoma. There should be histological confirmation of the disease.

T Clinical Classification

T – Primary Tumour

TX   Primary tumour cannot be assessed
T0   No evidence of primary tumour

T1   Tumour(s) of bulbar conjunctiva (Figs. 455, 456)

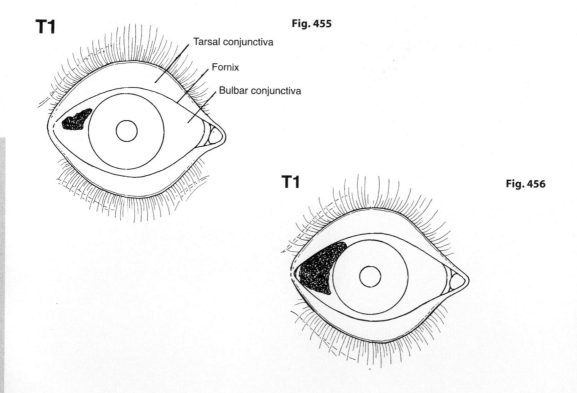

T1

Fig. 455

Tarsal conjunctiva

Fornix

Bulbar conjunctiva

T1

Fig. 456

T2   Tumour(s) of bulbar conjunctiva with corneal extension (Fig. 457)
T3   Tumour(s) extend(s) into conjunctival fornix, palpebral conjunctiva, or caruncle (Fig. 458)

T2

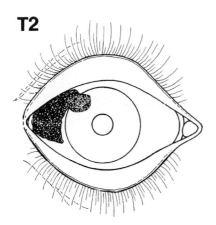

Fig. 457

T3

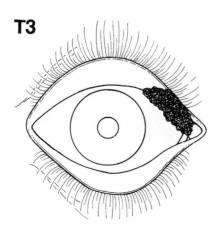

Fig. 458

▌T4   Tumour(s) invade(s) eyelid (Fig. 459), globe, orbit, sinuses, or central nervous system

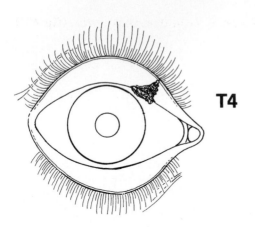

Fig. 459

T4

pT Pathological Classification

pT – Primary Tumour

pTX   Primary tumour cannot be assessed
pT0   No evidence of primary tumour
pT1   Tumour(s) of bulbar conjunctiva confined to the epithelium
pT2   Tumour(s) of bulbar conjunctiva occupying not more than 0.8 mm in thickness with invasion of the substantia propria (Fig. 460)

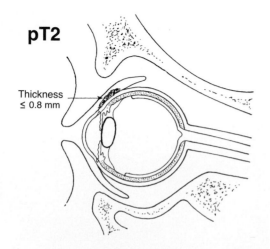

Fig. 460

pT2

Thickness
≤ 0.8 mm

pT3   Tumour(s) of bulbar conjunctiva more than 0.8 mm in thickness with invasion of the substantia propria or tumour(s) involving the palpebral or caruncular conjunctiva (Fig. 461)

pT4   Tumour(s) invade(s) eyelid, globe, orbit, sinuses, or central nervous system (Fig. 462)

pT3

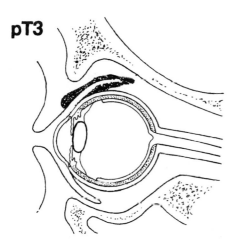

Fig. 461

pT4

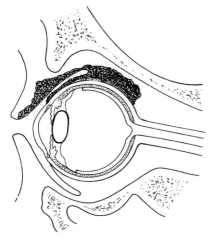

Fig. 462

Malignant Melanoma of Uvea (ICD-O C69.3, 4)

Rules for Classification

There should be histological confirmation of the disease.

Anatomical Sites

1. Iris (C69.4)
2. Ciliary body (C69.4)
3. Choroid (C69.3)

T Clinical Classification

T – Primary Tumour

TX   Primary tumour cannot be assessed
T0   No evidence of primary tumour

Iris

T1   Tumour limited to the iris
        T1a   not more than 3 clock hours in size (Fig. 463a,b)
        T1b   more than 3 clock hours in size (Fig. 464a,b)
        T1c   with melanomalytic glaucoma

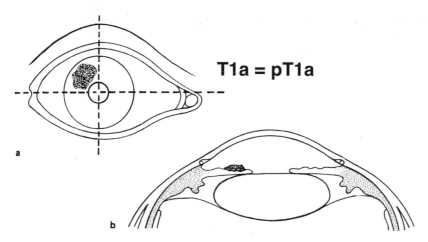

Fig. 463a, b

T1a = pT1a

a

b

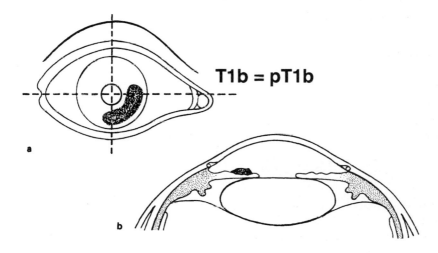

Fig. 464a, b

T1b = pT1b

a

b

T2   Tumour confluent with or extending into the ciliary body or chorioid (Fig. 465a,b)

      T2a   with melanomalytic glaucoma

T3   Tumour with scleral extension (Fig. 466a,b)

      T3a   Tumour with scleral extension and melanomalytic glaucoma

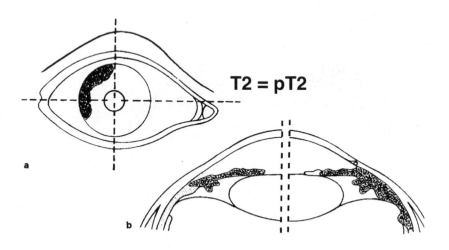

Fig. 465a, b

T2 = pT2

a

b

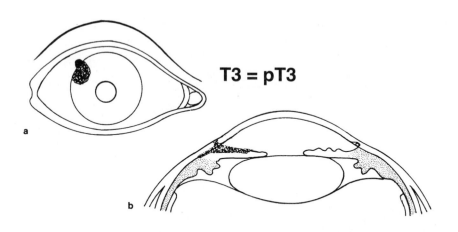

Fig. 466a, b

T3 = pT3

a

b

▌ T4   Tumour with extraocular extension (Fig. 467a,b)

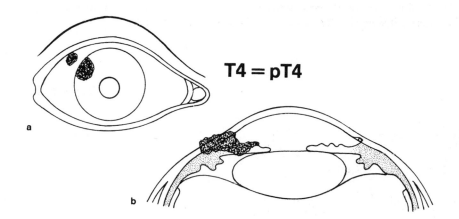

Fig. 467a, b

T4 = pT4

a

b

Ciliary Body and Choroid

T1   Tumour 10 mm or less at greatest diameter and 2.5 mm or less at greatest height (thickness) (Figs. 468, 469a,b)
    T1a   Without extraocular extension
    T1b   With microscopic extraocular extension
    T1c   With macroscopic extraocular extension

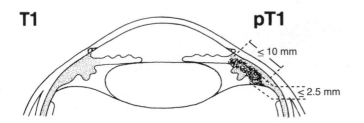

T1   **pT1**

≤ 10 mm

≤ 2.5 mm

Fig. 468

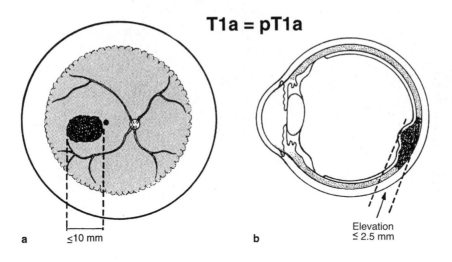

T1a = pT1a

Fig. 469a, b

a   ≤10 mm

b

Elevation
≤ 2.5 mm

T2   Tumour greater than 10 mm and not more than 16 mm at greatest diameter and more
      than 2.5 mm but not more than 10 mm at greatest height (Figs. 470, 471a,b)
      T2a   without extraocular extension
      T2b   with microscopic extraocular extension
      T2c   with macroscopic extraocular extension

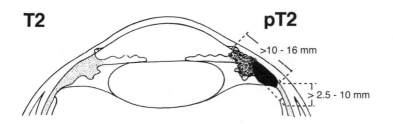

T2   **pT2**

>10 - 16 mm

> 2.5 - 10 mm

Fig. 470

T2 = pT2

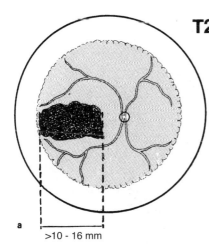

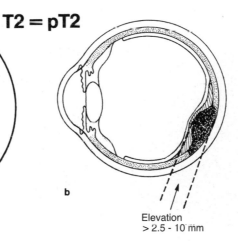

a

>10 - 16 mm

b

Elevation
> 2.5 - 10 mm

Fig. 471a, b

T3   Tumour more than 16 mm at greatest diameter and/or greater than 10 mm at greatest height, *without* extraocular extension (Figs. 472, 473a,b)

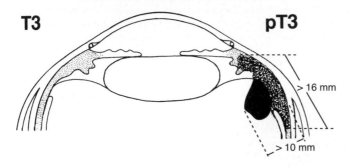

Fig. 472

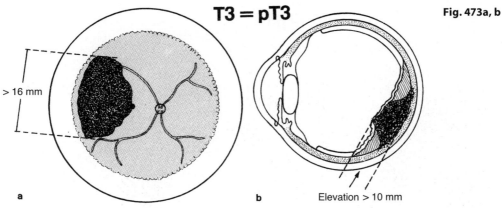

Fig. 473a, b

T4   Tumour more than 16 mm at greatest diameter and/or greater than 10 mm at greatest
       height *with* extraocular extension (Figs. 474, 475a,b)

Note
When basal diameter and apical height do not fit this classification, the largest tumour dimension should be
used for classification. In clinical practice, the tumour base may be estimated in optic disk diameters (dd)
(average: 1dd = 1.5 mm). The height may be estimated in diopters (average: 3 diopter = 1 mm). Techniques
such as ultrasonography are frequently used to provide more accurate measurements.

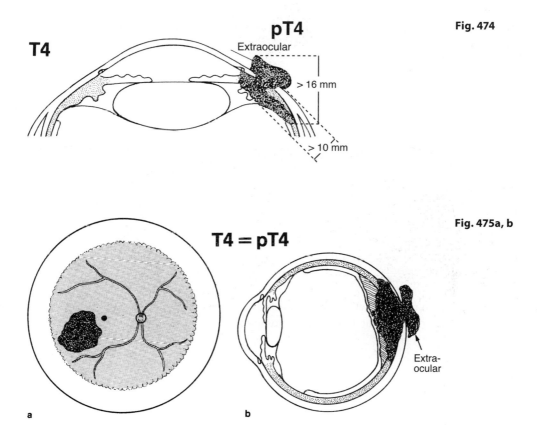

Fig. 474

Fig. 475a, b

pT Pathological Classification

The pT categories correspond to the T categories.

Retinoblastoma (ICD-O C69.2)

Rules for Classification

In bilateral cases, the eyes should be classified separately. The classification does not apply to complete spontaneous regression of the tumour. There should be histological confirmation of the disease in an enucleated eye.

T Clinical Classification

T – Primary Tumour

TX   Primary tumour cannot be assessed
T0   No evidence of primary tumour

T1   Tumour confined to the retina (No vitreous seeding or significant retinal detachment, or subretinal fluid over 5 mm from tumour base) (Fig. 476)
      T1a   Any eye in which the largest tumour is less than or equal to 3mm in height *and* no tumour is located closer than 1 DD (1.5 mm) to the optic nerve or fovea (Fig. 477a,b)
      T1b   All other eyes in which the tumour(s) are confined to the retina regardless of location or size (up to half the volume of the eye).

T1   **pT1**   **Fig. 476**

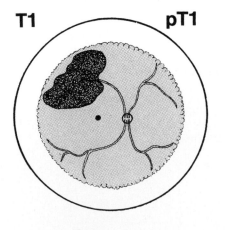

Retinoblastoma (side text)

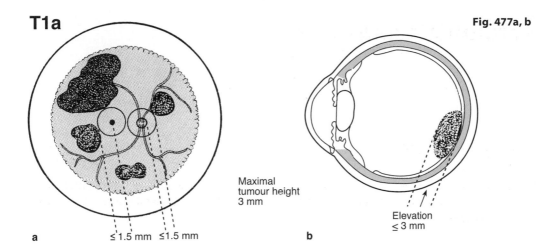

T1a

Maximal
tumour height
3 mm

Elevation
≤ 3 mm

a   ≤ 1.5 mm ≤ 1.5 mm   b

Fig. 477a, b

T2   Tumour with contiguous spread to adjacent tissues or spaces (vitreous or subretinal spaces)

T2a   Minimal tumour spread to vitreous and/or subretinal space. Fine local or diffuse vitreous seeding and/or serous retinal detachment up to total detachment may be present, but no clumps, lumps, snowballs or avascular masses in the vitreous or subretinal space. Calcium flecks in the vitreous or subretinal space are allowed. The tumour may fill up to 2/3 the volume of the eye (Fig. 478).

T2b   Massive tumour spread to vitreous and/or subretinal space. Vitreous seeding and/or subretinal implantation may consist of lumps, clumps, snowballs, or avascular tumour masses. Retinal detachment may be total. Tumour may fill up to 2/3 the volume of the eye (Fig. 479).

T2c   Unsalvageable intraocular disease. Tumour fills more than 2/3 the eye (Fig. 480) or there is no possibilty of visual rehabilitation or one or more of the following are present:
   – Tumour associated glaucoma, either neovascular or angle closure
   – Anterior segment extension of tumour
   – Ciliary body extension of tumour
   – Hyphema (significant)
   – Massive vitreous hemorrhage
   – Tumour in contact with lens
   – Orbital cellulitis-like presentation (massive tumour necrosis)

T2a

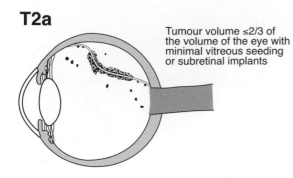

Tumour volume ≤2/3 of the volume of the eye with minimal vitreous seeding or subretinal implants

Fig. 478

T2b

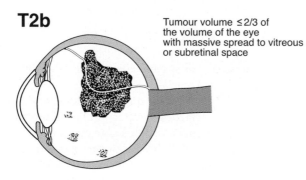

Tumour volume ≤ 2/3 of the volume of the eye with massive spread to vitreous or subretinal space

Fig. 479

T2c

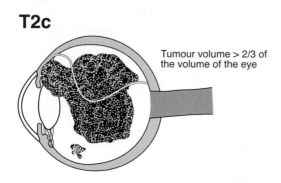

Tumour volume > 2/3 of the volume of the eye

Fig. 480

T3   Invasion of optic nerve and/or optic coats (Fig. 481a,b)
T4   Extraocular tumour (Fig. 482a,b)

Note
The suffix (m) may be added to the appropriate T categories to indicate multiple tumours, e.g., T2(m).

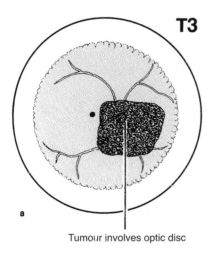

T3

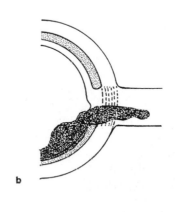

Fig. 481a, b

a

Tumour involves optic disc

b

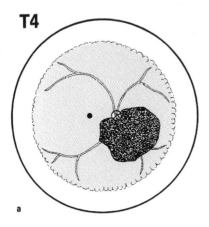

T4

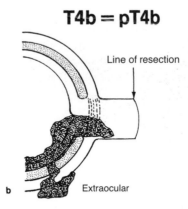

Fig. 482a, b

T4b = pT4b

Line of resection

a

b   Extraocular

pT Pathological Classification

pT – Primary Tumour

pTX   Primary tumour cannot be assessed

pT0   No evidence of primary tumour

pT1   Tumour confined to the retina, vitreous, or subretinal space. No optic nerve or choroidal invasion

pT2   Minimal invasion of the optic nerve and/or optic coats or focal invasion of choroid

    pT2a   Tumour invades optic nerve up to, but not through, the level of the lamina cribosa

    pT2b   Tumour invades choroid focally

    pT2c   Tumour invades optic nerve up to but not through the level of lamina cribrosa *and* invades the choroid focally

pT3   Significant invasion of the optic nerve or optic coats or massive invasion of choroid

    pT3a   Tumour invades optic nerve through the level of lamina cribrosa but not the line of resection

    pT3b   Tumour massively invades the choroid

    pT3c   Tumour invades the optic nerve through the level of the lamina cribrosa but not the line of resection *and* massively invades the choroid

pT4   Extraocular extension which includes any of the following:
- Invasion of optic nerve to the line of resection
- Invasion of orbit through the sclera
- Extension both anteriorly or posteriorly into the orbit
- Extension into the brain
- Extension into the subarachnoidal space of the optic nerve
- Extension to the apex of the orbit
- Extension to, but not through chiasm
- Extend into the brain beyond chiasm

Editors' Note

Today enucleation of an eye for retinoblastoma is a rare event. Therefore, we do not have not included figures for the pT categories.

Sarcoma of Orbit (ICD-O C69.6)

Rules for Classification

The classification applies only to sarcomas of soft tissue and bone. There should be histological confirmation of the disease and division of cases by histological type.

T Clinical Classification

T – Primary Tumour

TX   Primary tumour cannot be assessed
T0   No evidence of primary tumour

T1   Tumour 15 mm or less in greatest dimension (Fig. 483)
T2   Tumour more than 15 mm in greatest dimension without invasion of globe or bony wall (Fig. 484)
T3   Tumour of any size with invasion of orbital tissues and/or bony walls (Fig. 485)
T4   Tumour invades globe or periorbital structures such as: eyelids, temporal fossa, nasal cavity/paranasal sinuses, and/or central nervous system (Fig. 486)

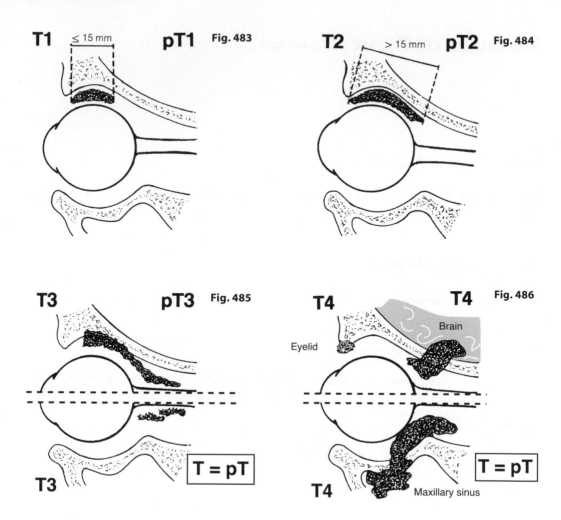

T1 ≤ 15 mm   **pT1** Fig. 483

T2 > 15 mm   **pT2** Fig. 484

T3   **pT3** Fig. 485

T3

T = pT

T4   **T4** Fig. 486

Eyelid

Brain

T4   Maxillary sinus

T = pT

pT Pathological Classification

The pT categories correspond to the T categories.

Carcinoma of Lacrimal Gland (ICD-O C69.5)

Rules for Classification

There should be histological confirmation of the disease and division of cases by histological type.

T Clinical Classification

T – Primary Tumour

TX   Primary tumour cannot be assessed
T0   No evidence of primary tumour

T1   Tumour 2.5 cm or less in greatest dimension, limited to the lacrimal gland (Fig. 487a, b)
T2   Tumour more than 2.5 cm, but not more than 5.0 cm, in greatest dimension, limited to the lacrimal gland (Fig. 488a, b)

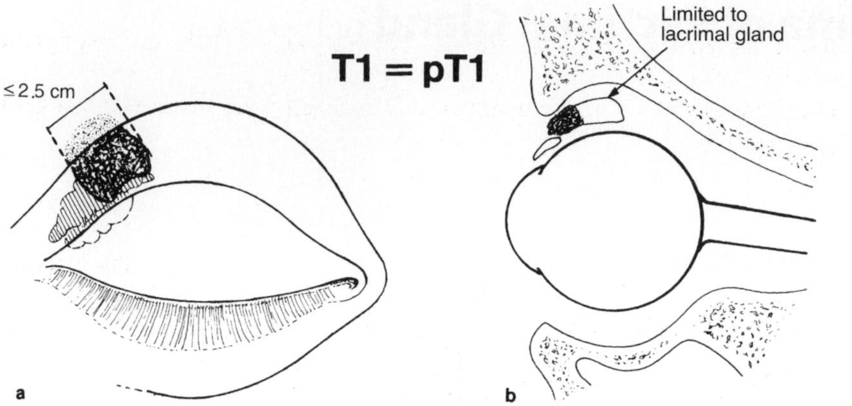

Carcinoma of Lacrimal Gland

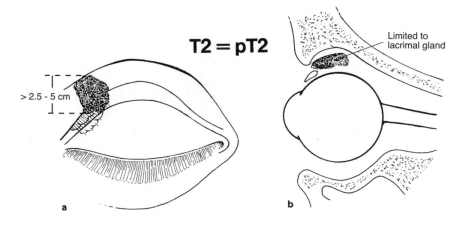

T1 = pT1

≤ 2.5 cm

Limited to
lacrimal gland

a   b

Fig. 487a, b

T2 = pT2

> 2.5 - 5 cm

Limited to
lacrimal gland

a   b

Fig. 488a,b

T3   Tumour invades periosteum
    T3a   Tumour not more than 5.0 cm, invades the periosteum of the lacrimal gland
           fossa (Fig. 489a,b)
    T3b   Tumour more than 5.0 cm in greatest dimension with periosteal invasion
           (Fig. 490a,b)

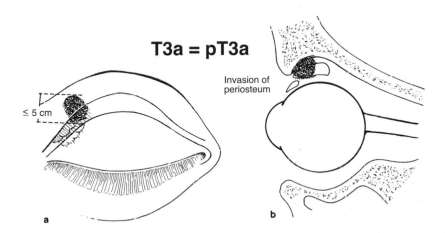

Fig. 489a, b

T3a = pT3a

Invasion of
periosteum

≤ 5 cm

a   b

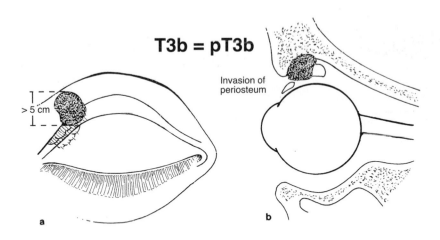

Fig. 490a, b

T3b = pT3b

Invasion of
periosteum

> 5 cm

a   b

T4   Tumour invades the orbital soft tissues, optic nerve, or globe with or without bone invasion; tumour extends beyond the orbit to adjacent structures including brain (Figs. 491, 492)

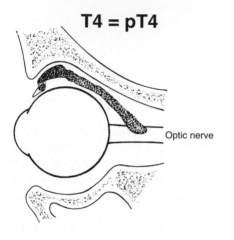

T4 = pT4

Fig. 491

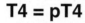

Optic nerve

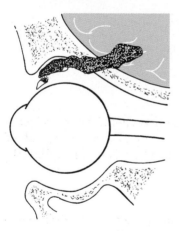

T4 = pT4

Fig. 492

pT Pathological Classification

The pT categories correspond to the T categories.

Hodgkin Lymphoma

Introductory Notes

At the present time it is not considered practical to propose a TNM classification for Hodgkin lymphoma.

Following the development of the Ann Arbor classification for Hodgkin lymphoma in 1971, the significance of two important observations with major impact on staging has been appreciated. First, extralymphatic disease, if localized and related to adjacent lymph node disease, does not adversely affect the survival of patients. Secondly, laparotomy with splenectomy has been introduced as a method of obtaining more information on the extent of the disease within the abdomen[1].

A stage classification based on information from histopathological examination of the spleen and lymph nodes obtained at laparotomy cannot be compared with another without such exploration. Therefore, two systems of classification are presented, a clinical (cS) and a pathological (pS).

Editor's note
[1] The same is valid for staging by laparoscopy.

Clinical Staging (cS)

Although recognized as incomplete, this is easily performed and should be reproducible from one centre to another. It is determined by history, clinical examination, imaging, blood analysis, and the initial biopsy report. Bone marrow biopsy must be taken from a clinically or radiologically non-involved area of bone.

Liver Involvement
Clinical evidence of liver involvement must include either enlargement of the liver and at least an abnormal serum alkaline phosphatase level and two different liver function test abnormalities, or an abnormal liver demonstrated by imaging and one abnormal liver function test.

Spleen Involvement
Clinical evidence of spleen involvement is accepted if there is palpable enlargement of the spleen confirmed by imaging.

Lymphatic and Extralymphatic Disease

The lymphatic structures are as follows:
- Lymph nodes
- Waldeyer ring
- Spleen
- Appendix
- Thymus
- Peyer patches

The lymph nodes are grouped into regions and one or more (2, 3, etc.) may be involved. The spleen is designated S and extralymphatic organs or sites E.

Lung Involvement

Lung involvement limited to one lobe, or perihilar extension associated with ipsilateral lymphadenopathy, or unilateral pleural effusion with or without lung involvement but with hilar lymphadenopathy is considered as localized extralymphatic disease.

Liver Involvement

Liver involvement is always considered as diffuse extralymphatic disease.

Pathological Staging (pS)

This takes into account additional data and has a higher degree of precision. It should be applied whenever possible. A – (minus) or + (plus) sign should be added to the various symbols for the examined tissues, depending on the results of histopathological examination.

Histopathological Information

This is classified by symbols indicating the tissue sampled. The following notation is common to the distant metastases (or M1 categories) of all regions classified by the TNM system. However, in order to conform with the Ann Arbor classification, the initial letters used in that system are also given.

Pulmonary	PUL or L	Bone marrow	MAR or M
Osseous	OSS or O	Pleura	PLE or P
Hepatic	HEP or H	Peritoneum	PER
Brain	BRA	Adrenals	ADR
Lymph nodes	LYM or N	Skin	SKI or D
Others	OTH		

Clinical Stages (cS)

Stage I   Involvement of a single lymph node region (I) (Figs. 493–496), or localized involvement of a single extralymphatic organ or site (I_E) (Fig. 497)

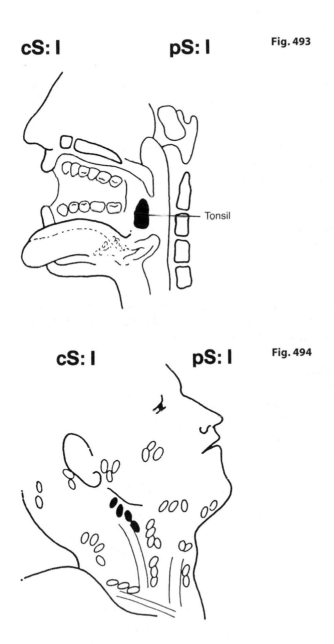

cS: I   **pS: I**   **Fig. 493**

Tonsil

cS: I   **pS: I**   **Fig. 494**

cS: I$_S$ pS: I$_S$

Fig. 495

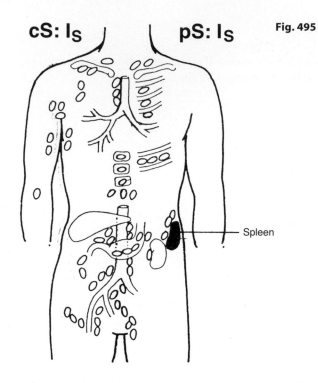

Spleen

cS: I = pS: I

Fig. 496a, b

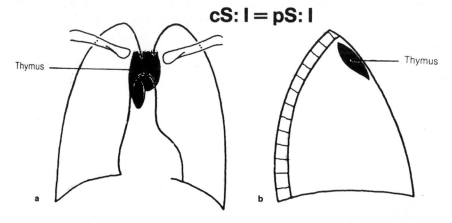

Thymus

Thymus

a   b

Hodgkin Lymphoma

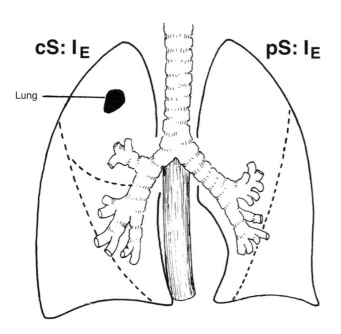

Fig. 497

Stage II   Involvement of two or more lymph node regions on the same side of the dia-
            phragm (II$_5$) (Fig. 498), or localized involvement of a single extralymphatic or-
            gan or site and its regional lymph node(s) with or without involvement of other
            lymph node regions on the same side of the diaphragm (II$_E$) (Fig. 499)

Note
The number of lymph node regions involved may be indicated by a subscript (e.g., II3).

cS: II₅   pS: II₅   Fig. 498

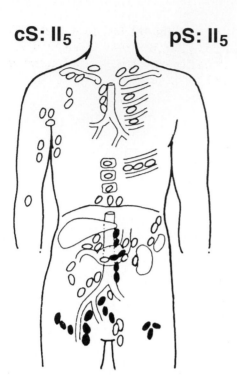

cS: II_E   pS: II_E   Fig. 499

Lung ——

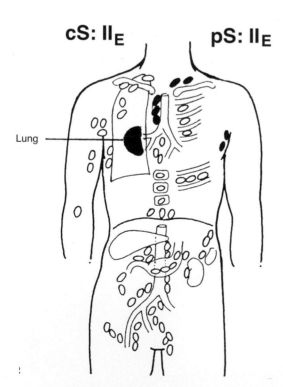

Stage III   Involvement of lymph node regions on both sides of the diaphragm (III) (Fig. 500), which may also be accompanied by localized involvement of an associated extralymphatic organ or site (III_E) (Fig. 501a-c), or by involvement of the spleen (III_S), or both (III_{E+S}) (Fig. 502a,b)

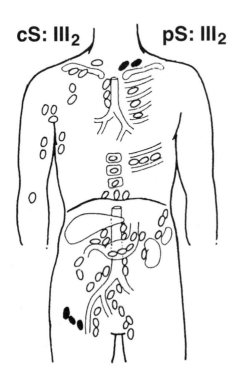

cS: III_2 pS: III_2 Fig. 500

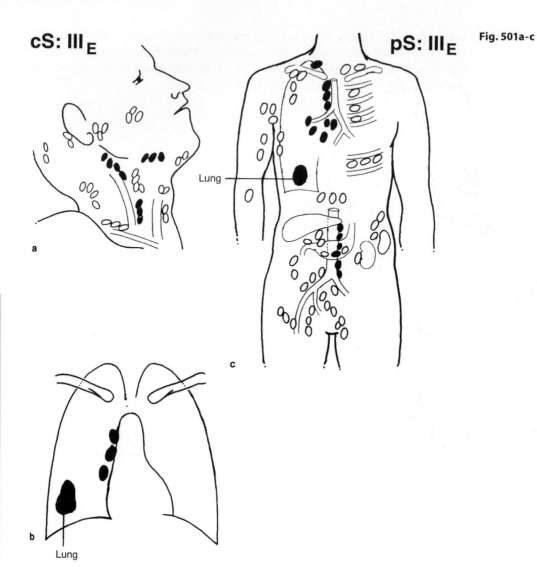

cS: III$_E$

pS: III$_E$

Fig. 501a-c

Lung

a

b   Lung

c

cS: III $_{E+S}$

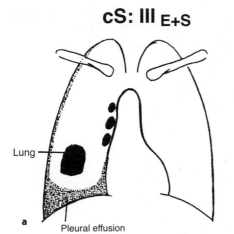

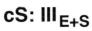

Fig. 502a, b

Lung

a

Pleural effusion

cS: III $_{E+S}$

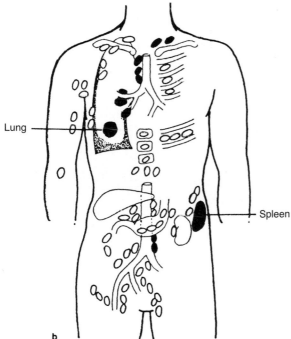

Lung

Spleen

b

Stage IV   Disseminated (multifocal) involvement of one or more extralymphatic organs, with or without associated lymph node involvement (Figs. 503–504) or isolated extralymphatic organ involvement with distant (non-regional) nodal involvement (Fig. 505)

Note
The site of Stage IV disease is identified further by specifying sites according to the notations listed above.

cS: IV(LYM, HEP) pS: IV(LYM, HEP)

Fig. 503

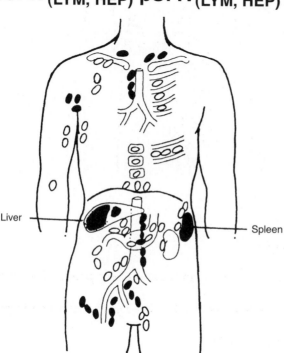

Liver

Spleen

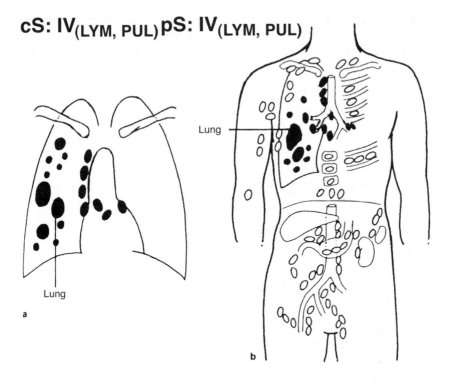

cS: IV$_{(LYM, PUL)}$ pS: IV$_{(LYM, PUL)}$

Fig. 504a, b

A and B Classification (Symptoms)

Each stage should be divided into A and B according to the absence or presence of defined general symptoms. These are:
1. Unexplained weight loss of more than 10% of the usual body weight in the 6 months prior to first attendance
2. Unexplained fever with temperature above 38° C
3. Night sweats

Note
Pruritus alone does not qualify for B classification nor does a short, febrile illness associated with a known infection.

cS: IV_(LYM,HEP) pS: IV_(LYM,HEP)

Fig. 505

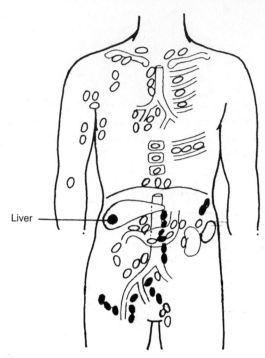

Liver

Pathological Stages (pS)

The definitions of the four stages follow the same criteria as the clinical stages but with the additional information obtained following laparotomy or laparoscopy (see note p. 371). Splenectomy, liver biopsy, lymph node biopsy, and marrow biopsy are mandatory for the establishment of pathological stages. The results of these biopsies are recorded as indicated above (see p. 372).

Hodgkin Lymphoma

Non-Hodgkin Lymphoma

As in Hodgkin lymphoma, at the present time it is not considered practical to propose a TNM classification for Non-Hodgkin lymphomas. Since no other convincing and tested staging system is available, the Ann Arbor classification is recommended with the same modification as for Hodgkin lymphoma (see Figs. 493–505, pp. 372ff.).

Printing: Krips bv, Meppel, The Netherlands
Binding: Stürtz, Würzburg, Germany